The Other Side of the Valley

Healing Through Altered States of Consciousness

The Other Side
of the Valley

Healing Through Altered States
of Consciousness

Linda M. D. Edwards Ph.D

BOOKS

Winchester, UK
Washington, USA

First published by O-Books, 2019
O-Books is an imprint of John Hunt Publishing Ltd., 3 East St., Alresford,
Hampshire SO24 9EE, UK
office1@jhpbooks.net
www.johnhuntpublishing.com

For distributor details and how to order please visit the 'Ordering' section on our website.

ISBN: 978 1 78099 826 8
978 1 78099 825 1 (ebook)
Library of Congress Control Number: 2015937453

A CIP catalogue record for this book is available from the British Library.

Design: Stuart Davies

Printed and bound by CPI Group (UK) Ltd, Croydon, CR0 4YY, UK

We operate a distinctive and ethical publishing philosophy in
all areas of our business, from our global network of authors to
production and worldwide distribution.

Contents

Chapter I

Introduction

I have been on a profound journey of self-awareness and self-healing over the last eighteen years as I have studied and researched as much as I could about altered states of consciousness (ASCs) and healing. I have been very privileged to experience all of the ASCs discussed in this book. Some of these experiences remain unfathomable to my logical mind; and yet, I have felt the very real benefits on the mental, emotional, and physical levels.

My concept of life has been changed forever. I am no longer sceptical of the inexplicable, however, far from accepting all of these concepts without question, I remain curious about the potential of using ASCs to achieve desired change. I know that in this work I have merely uncovered the 'tip of the iceberg' and that this is the beginning of a lifelong quest to uncover more. Based on what I have discovered so far, it appears that as human beings, we have forgotten more than we can remember. We have become so involved with the material world that we have forgotten much of our innate nature, and hence many forms of healing that we can access through ASCs.

I started this journey as a fearful sceptic, someone who was afraid of any form of consciousness other than that which I used on a daily logical basis. I had originally trained in western allopathic medicine to be a podiatrist. However, by the age of 27 I had climbed to the top of my career ladder in this field and I was bored. So I explored other alternatives and by my early thirties had become a Chief Executive in the British National Health Service. To me, at that time, allowing myself to go into trance was akin to giving away my power to someone or even worse, something unknown. I was trapped in a web of reality where only the tangible and knowable was real, and even then, only when it could be scientifically proven.

My initial explorations into ASCs were through hypnosis where my intent had been to prove that this 'stuff' would never be able to work with me. I had an iron grip on my conscious mind, and was far removed from my emotional and physical self; yet, something inside prompted me to start this exploration into the unknown, albeit under rather false pretences. I realise now that in order to get me to the point of embarkation, my conscious mind needed to feel safe. Little did I know how this would change my life so dramatically.

The journey so far, has taken eighteen years, and despite all I have learned, I still feel like a novice stepping into a world of the unknown. The more I learn, the more I realise how little I really know. It is my intention that this book, my experiences, and conclusions will help inform others about the benefits of entering into ASCs in order to facilitate their own health and well-being.

Linda Edwards 2012

Chapter II

Understanding Trance and Altered States of Consciousness

Trance is often wrapped up in the mystique of eastern philosophy, and even the occult. It is seen as something mysterious and strange to be avoided at all costs. What many people do not know is that trance or altered states of consciousness (ASC) are naturally occurring states in our everyday existence. Some people have a greater conscious awareness or control over these states, however, despite our lack of awareness most of us will experience a new state every ninety seconds or so.

So what is it about trance or ASC (these terms will be used synonymously throughout this text) that causes so much anxiety and even fear in many people? In my experience, I would say that this fear is based on a lack of knowledge, a fear of the unknown, and a fear of things that appear intangible. This is the point at which I started on my own journey into understanding trance. I was ignorant about anything other than the tangible, 'provable' things in life. I thought if you couldn't physically see it, hear it, feel it or scientifically prove 'it' then 'it' could not exist. However, my curiosity was piqued as I began to unfold through experience with the 'non-seeable' often non-scientifically provable aspects of life. I soon became enthralled and excited about the full potential of life, combining the seen with the unseen. This segment of the paper is an exploration of the question, 'What is trance?' It delves into recent research about ASC, and unfolds my own learnings and their impact on my life, and those I have worked with.

What Is Trance?

The advance of quantum physics and the work of neuro scientists over the last few decades are beginning to shine some light on the hitherto dark area of our other than conscious awareness. Trance and altered states of consciousness enable us to access the great repository of our knowing that is other than conscious. A statement frequently used in the scientific community is that 20 per cent of our mind is conscious, and 80 per cent is unconscious, however, this is yet to be proven. Nonetheless, it is evident that in our usual up-time state of consciousness we only have access to a portion of available 'information'. So, the theory is that by beginning to train ourselves to enter ASCs with volition we are increasing the amount of consciousness available to us.

What Is the Difference between Our Conscious and Unconscious Mind?

The work of brain researcher Benjamin Libet (2004), suggests that the conscious mind will not actually initiate an act, but will select and control the outcome. He states that other research indicates that although the conscious mind has a limited capacity, it excels in context sensitivity, internal consistency and serial processing. (It has been suggested by several scientists that conscious mind overload lies behind a number of psychotic illnesses.) The unconscious mind, on the other hand, is capable of engaging in diverse and highly specialised tasks, which may even be contradictory to one another.

An analogy that clarifies the relationship between the conscious and unconscious aspects of our mind is one of the captain of a ship (*Overdurf & Silverthorn, 1994*). The conscious mind is the captain, setting the course or direction. Whereas, the unconscious aspect of the mind is like the crew of the ship whose job is to carry out the captain's orders.

Can We Actually Measure Consciousness in the Brain?

Medical science is now able to measure consciousness as a gauge of the brain's activity. Currently four levels of brain-wave activity have been defined, each designated a Greek letter: Alpha, Beta, Theta and Delta (*Marsolek*, 2003). These can be identified and measured by an electroencephalogram (EEG) machine.

Alpha waves: are present in the 'resting state' of the brain. This is a passive state where we are relaxed and non-critical. An example of this state is when we are relaxing and listening to music. In this state we are aware of external stimuli. So-called, 'Mystical states of consciousness' occur in this state. They usually occur prior to, and just after falling sleep. This 'Alpha State' occurs voluntarily during light hypnosis, meditation, biofeedback, daydreaming, hypnogogic (the transition from waking to sleeping) and hypnopompic (the transition from sleeping to waking) states. These brain waves range from 8 to 13 cycles per second.

Beta waves: are present in our normal waking state of consciousness. About 75 per cent of our waking consciousness is generally occupied with monitoring our body's physical functions. The remaining 25 per cent is occupied with thinking and planning activities. These brain waves range from 14 to 27 cycles per second.

Theta waves: occur when we are in a state of reverie, a level of consciousness that is open to intuition and inspiration. When we are at this level of consciousness, stimuli are quite often ignored. Theta naturally occurs during light sleep. It is also accessed during biofeedback and meditation. At this level of consciousness, we are usually unaware of our surroundings. These brain waves range from 4 to 8 cycles per second.

Delta Waves: is the lowest level of brain activity. This state usually occurs during deep sleep when we are unreceptive to any stimuli.

These four levels of brain-wave activity have enabled scientists to understand the various components of consciousness.

What Are Altered States of Consciousness?

Medical science and psychology have determined that we experience vast numbers of altered states of consciousness in our everyday life. We often experience daydreaming, meditation, the internal scanning of our inner states, happiness, excitement, depression or sadness, as well as the normal waking state, sleep, and dreaming, and the states in between.

All ASCs are simply deviations from our normal consciousness; however, many people have an impression of trance that is based on their limited knowledge of altered states of consciousness. These are usually based on stage hypnosis or seeing mystics who look as if they are 'zoned' out. For several hundred years Western society has distrusted these states and the people practising them. These days such people are often deemed as crack pots or 'weirdoes'. It is as if even talking about such things is too frightening for most people to even consider. However, this view is beginning to change with an increasing number of neuroscientists, physicists, psychologists, and psychiatrists, other medical doctors, and parapsychologists beginning to understand how these types of phenomena work, and whether or not they have value.

An altered state of consciousness (ASC or trance) is generally defined as any mental state that is perceived by an individual, or an observer, as being significantly different from 'normal' waking consciousness. These ASCs may range from ordinary daydreams to encounters of near death experiences (also known as NDEs), or apparently mystical occurrences. From personal experience, we can tell when we are in an ASC when we experience any of the following: marked alterations in our thinking, a distortion of time, apparent loss of control, changes in emotional state, and changes in how we perceive our body either in sensations or our body image and other perceptual distortions.

The following diagram shows some ASCs depicted on two axes, mind expansion or dissociation, and gain or loss of control.

(Inge-Heinze, 1984)

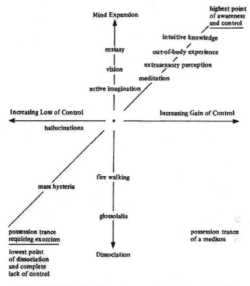

Figure 1: The levels of consciousness demonstrated in ASCs

Figure 1: The levels of consciousness demonstrated in ASCs

Charles Tart, (2000) a great proponent of understanding ASC from simple trance states to out of body experiences (OBEs), suggests that our supposed normal consciousness should in fact be called the 'consensus trance'. The body of knowledge known as NLP (Neuro Linguistic Programming) also supports this point of view, stating that we perceive our reality as a construct of our beliefs and cultural conditioning. Tart further says that at any time we perceive a belief as absolute or unchangeable we are actually in a trance. This may explain why we have so much difficulty in understanding trance and ASC, because we are continually moving in and out of various ASCs. Both advocates and sceptics of the value of these states are often deeply entrenched in their 'beliefs', creating a vast schism between two opposing viewpoints. This is something I encounter quite often when these topics somehow slide into social conversations. As a student of trance, and someone who has had many positive experiences of induced ASCs, I am continually amazed at how fearful many sceptics are when I subtly, and sometimes, not so subtly, challenge their beliefs. However, I do believe that there are simple ways to enable people to understand trance to remove their fears.

Neurologists traditionally feel that all that we see, hear, feel and think is created in, or mediated by the brain. Some neurologists are also attempting to determine if there are any neurological origins to spiritual and mystical experiences. In his work, Dr. Andrew Newberg, (2002) has been mapping the brains of meditators in mystical states. He has used radioactive tracers that are pumped into the brain at these specific moments and 'photographed.' What he found most noticeable was that the 'quieter' areas of the brain really stood out. He states, 'A bundle of neurons in the superior parietal lobe, toward the top and back of the brain, had gone dark.' This part of the brain requires sensory input to function and is called the 'orientation association area'. This area enables us to know where we are in time and space. When our orientation association area quietens down in certain ASCs, we actually lose the distinction between ourselves and the rest of the world. We then perceive everything as self, totally interwoven and connected.

This activity, or lack thereof, shows us how brain function is related to our mental-emotional states. This has stimulated a number of people to ask if this means that the experience of these altered states is mechanical. So, given this, let us consider what would happen if we were able to photograph our brain whilst we were eating a banana. The neurological activity in the brain would not simply negate the reality of the banana. Newberg says, 'There is no way to determine whether the neurological changes associated with spiritual experience mean that the brain is causing those experiences... or is instead perceiving a spiritual reality.'

In his work dating back to the early 1970s, researcher, Michael Persinger of Laurentian University in Canada (1987), used a device to send a weak magnetic field into people's heads to influence their temporal lobes. This can be seen to create experiences described as mystical or OBEs. In one of his studies for example, a woman who was experiencing nightly visitations by the 'holy spirit', sadly found that these were caused by a clock on her bedside table. The 'magnetic pulses generated by the clock (were) similar to shapes that evoke electrical seizures in epileptic rats and sensitive humans.'

In another experiment a journalist who had previously experienced a 'haunting', reported 'rushes of fear' and a visual apparition, which he said was very similar to his original experiences. Persinger suggested that this type of experiment may help researchers to understand the environmental variables that give rise to the original occurrences of this kind of phenomena. He later correlated experiences attributed to Christ and Mary at Marmora, Ontario, Canada, to the location of an open pit magnetite mine that had been filling with water. He was able to identify that the epicentres for local seismic events had also moved closer to the pit. He said, 'Most of the messages attributed to spiritual beings by "sensitive" individuals occurred one or two days after increased global geomagnetic activity.' This research would indicate that there could be a potential causal, non-paranormal explanation for some spiritual experiences. Other researchers believe that when areas of the brain, such as the orientation area, become quiet, it is a regression from higher functioning to a more primitive, unthinking, yet aware state.

Laurence O. McKinney author of *Neurotheology: Virtual Religion in the 21st Century* (1994) writes that the state of 'selfless perception would be experienced as a state of grace to a religious Westerner, and Samadhi or Satori to a Hindu or a Buddhist.' However, he then goes on to say that this self-induced state is a 'lower consciousness, in fact.' McKinney states that he believes that these occurrences can be positive, that 'moments of mild ego loss are instructive, not destructive, because they were done purposefully... Every time we repeat thoughtfully something that we love to do, we add to our growing networks of associative energy.'

Neuroscientist Rhawn Joseph raises the question, 'Are these states a regression to a more primitive functioning that is only beneficial because it's managed by the "higher" consciousness of normal cognitive functioning?' Rhawn is author of *The Right Brain and the Unconscious: Discovering the Stranger Within* (1992). He further questions assumptions such as, 'Why would the limbic system evolve specialized neurons or neural networks... to experience or hallucinate spirits, angels, and the souls of the living and the departed if these entities had no basis in reality? We can hear because there are sounds that can be perceived and because we evolved specialized brain tissue that analyzes this information. First came sounds, and then later, specialized nerve cells evolved that could analyze vibrations and then later, sounds. Likewise, if there were nothing to contemplate visually we would not have evolved eyes or visual cortex, which analyzes this information. Visual stimuli existed before the neurons that evolved in order to process these signs. Should not the same evolutionary principles apply to the limbic system and religious experience?'

Neurosurgeon, Wilder Penfield's (1978) research has significantly increased our understanding of the relationship between the brain and the mind. In his work with epileptics, he discovered that since the brain has no pain receptors, he could directly stimulate the brain of a conscious patient. One experiment that he carried out was to stimulate specific spots on the brain. He discovered that by stimulating one specific spot he would cause the person's arm to move, and when he then stimulated another spot they would suddenly smell lemons.

Penfield carried out numerous experiments that showed how specific experiences were located in different areas of the brain. His research, however, failed to show where and indeed if, the mind resided in the brain. He finally concluded that whilst all his experiments had been built on the principle that the brain generates the mind they in fact proved exactly the opposite.

In his recent publication, *The Open Focus Brain: Harnessing the Power of Attention to Heal Mind and Body* (2007), Dr. Les Fehmi, (a psychologist and neuro feedback researcher from Princeton) talks about the value of subjective experience along with what we know about the physical mechanisms in the brain. He describes an, 'open focus' state of awareness, which is signified by synchronous alpha frequencies in the brain. He initially experienced these alpha frequencies for himself thinking he had failed, he states; 'At the moment of surrender I experienced a deep and profound feeling of disappointment. Fortunately, I surrendered while still connected to my EEG and while still receiving feedback. It was surprising to observe that I now produced five times the amount of alpha than before the act of surrendering.' After learning how to open his focus and create the alpha waves, he said that he 'felt more open, lighter, freer, more energetic and spontaneous. A broader perspective ensued which allowed me to experience a more whole and subtle understanding. As the letting go unfolded, I felt more intimate with sensory experience, more intuitive...'

Fehmi found that he could force his brain to stop grasping, and move into open focus by utilizing this imagining space. He experienced this as a huge three-dimensional space, a space of nothingness, total silence, and timelessness. He noted that our attention is expanded and experienced with greater raptness, a sense of presence along with a centred and unified awareness. This is very similar to what meditators report when they quiet the orientation area in their brains. We can experience open focus quite simply ourselves by becoming aware of the space in between the letters on this page while we are attending to the words and the meanings of the words. We can also become aware of the space between us, and the computer screen, whilst at the same time become aware of sounds around us. Then, we let all of that stay with us as we attend to the words, and the meanings of the words, we read.

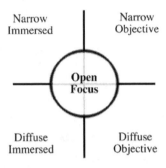

Figure 2: Various states of attention, showing where open focus resides.

The diagram depicted above is taken from the work of Les Fehmi. It shows a common attention style in each corner with what he calls the Open Focus State at the centre. This enables equal access to all attention modalities.

Dr Fehmi believes that the way we pay attention is fundamentally important. He has shown that if someone is always in narrow objective focus they will start to experience stress, regardless of the content of their attention. This is also supported by Huna, the spiritual beliefs of the ancient Hawaiians (see section on Huna). Fehmi himself, like many of us in today's society was persistently in narrow focus. He finally 'gave up' on his narrow focus and had a spontaneous breakthrough, finding himself in the open focus state. After studying this way of being, Fehmi now feels that much of the rampant use of drugs and the fascination with meditation and ecstatic and mystical states is in fact, due to Western society's chronic narrow focus. These ways of living, give the illusion of alleviating the tension of actually being in the chronic and narrow focus of 'consensus trance' or consensual reality.

The sense of feeling good that comes when we alter our attention and our consciousness has been shown to relieve many stress symptoms such as chronic pain and insomnia, along with skin and eye disorders. This has been demonstrated in the study of Transcendental Meditation, hypnotic trances and Fehmi's open focus. People, (including myself) who have been living their lives in 'narrow focus' often experience the most profound results. It has also been shown by Fehmi's work (along with others), that with regular practice most people will experience lasting changes.

Despite the fact that many of these changes are subjective, and hence currently relatively difficult to measure, some studies are showing how the focus of our attention may physically change the brain. For example neuroscientist, Susan Greenfield (2002) has shown how the hippocampi in London taxi drivers were enlarged proportionately to the length of their employment. She suggests that this may be related to their remembering abilities, as they learn more routes for negotiating London traffic. She also noted a similar study where just practising simple five-finger piano exercises for five days enhanced the area of the brain relating to the fingers. Furthermore, and more remarkably, she demonstrated that simply imagining the movements also created a comparable change in the brain, producing a measurable physical change. This adds to the accumulating body of knowledge that is beginning to prove that it is irrelevant whether something is 'real' or imagined, because our brain will respond in the same way.

As science is now acquiring the evidence to demonstrate that imagination itself changes the structure in the brain, it becomes more credible that an altered state can generate other paranormal phenomena. This adds further scientific credence to the ability to control pain demonstrated by people in and after hypnosis. This ability is increasingly being acknowledged as a natural, though seldom used, potential of the mind-body connection.

Parapsychologists Russell Targ and Jane Katra (1999), in their work on non-local consciousness and spiritual healing, state that the interconnectedness demonstrated in quantum physics is the explanation for people to be able to have the ability to undertake remote viewing and distant healing. When we do this we are connecting with the experience and 'knowingness' of oneness, a state of no separation. The nub of this is that separateness, be it mind and body, time and space, or self and others is nothing more than an illusion (something the mystics have been telling us for millennia). This has lead Targ and Katra to suggest that meditation and other consciousness altering practices may be more psychologically and physiologically powerful than we have hitherto believed. They say, 'The choice of where we put our attention is ultimately our most powerful freedom. Our choice of attitude and focus affects not only our own perceptions and experiences, but also the experiences and behaviours of others.'

We each go through many trances during our normal waking days, using our attention to alter our awareness, and by becoming aware of this we can all have a sense of how easy it is to shift our consciousness. These experiences may seem totally unlike the altered states seen in a shaman or someone in a hypnotic trance; however, it is simply a matter of degree.

In my experience, once people begin to understand the value of these daily light states of trance they become more open to experiencing other deeper states of consciousness. The deeper levels of trance used by shamans for healing are discussed in more detail later in this work. Suffice to know at this stage that reputable scientists like Edison and Einstein were known to use their abilities to go into natural trance states for creative breakthroughs. Einstein even said that he derived some of his formulae from, 'psychical entities as more or less clear images'

(1996).

Many people, who regularly practise meditation, hypnosis, and 'open focus' report, that they feel more in control of their lives. They often say that accessing these states gives them the ability to loosen the grip that 'consensus trance' has on their minds. A century ago William James (*James, 2003*) said, '...the mystical feeling of enlargement, union and emancipation has no specific intellectual content whatsoever of its own... We have no right, therefore, to invoke its prestige as distinctly in favor of any special belief.'

Physiological changes and disturbances can also produce ASCs, these include: hypoglycaemia, either spontaneous or subsequent to fasting (used by many traditional cultures such as when on a Vision Quest); hyperglycaemia (e.g. lethargy following a meal); dehydration (which are often partially responsible for the mental aberrations encountered on the desert or at sea); thyroid and adrenal gland dysfunctions; sleep deprivation; hyperventilation; narcolepsy; temporal lobe seizures (e.g. dreamy states and déja vu phenomena); and auras preceding a migraine or an epileptic seizure. A toxic delirium, which is another form of ASC, may be produced by fever, the ingestion of toxins, or the abrupt withdrawal from addictive drugs, such as alcohol and barbiturates. In addition, ASCs may be induced through the use of plant medicine and our Western everyday pharmaceutical drugs, such as anaesthetics, and the use of psychedelic, narcotic, sedative, and stimulant drugs.

William James (2003) puts this beautifully when he describes the subjective experiences associated with alcohol induced ASCs. 'One of the charms of drunkenness,' he writes, 'unquestionably lies in the deepening sense of reality and truth which is gained therein. In whatever light things may then appear to us, they seem more utterly what they are, more 'utterly utter' than when we are sober.'

ASCs in Healing.

Tart (2000) and Hebb (2002) describe the major role that healing through ASCs has played throughout history. The induction of these states has been used in almost every possible conceivable aspect of psychological therapy. For instance, shamans in many parts of the world will often go into trance or possession states in order to diagnose their patients' illnesses or to gain knowledge about a specific remedy or healing practice. Often, during the actual treatment or healing ceremony, the shaman, may view the production of an ASC in the patient as a crucial prerequisite for healing. There are many instances of healing practices throughout the world, and in different cultures that are specifically designed to take advantage of the suggestibility, increased meaning, tendency for emotional breakthrough, and the feelings of rejuvenation associated with ASCs.

The role of ASCs in treatment is evident through the ages from the early Egyptian and Greek practices of 'incubation' in their sleep temples to the current day faith cures at Lourdes and other religious shrines, the healing through prayer and meditation, the various methods of healing through touch, encounters with religious relics, spiritual healing, spirit possession cures, exorcism, mesmeric or magnetic treatment, right through to modern day hypnotherapy.

Both chemical and natural drugs can be used to induce ASCs for the purpose of healing. Other specific effects of ASCs in treatment are the non-specific effects of changes in consciousness in the maintenance of psychic equilibrium and health. For example, sleep and dreaming seem to serve important biological and psychological functions for us. ASC is also associated with sexual orgasm, and acts as a manifestation of many human desires as well as its obvious function in the survival of our species.

ASCs in Acquiring Knowledge.

ASCs are often used in an effort to gain inspiration, or some new knowledge or experience. Using the vehicle of religion, concentrated prayer, passive meditation, mystical and transcendental experiences, and divination states we have been able to open up new realms of possibility, reaffirm our moral values, resolve emotional conflicts, and even enable us to find better ways of functioning in the world. It is also important to recognize that among many indigenous cultures, spirit possession is believed to impart a superhuman knowledge, which could not possibly be gained during waking consciousness.

ASCs seem to enrich our experiences in many other ways, such as: the intense feelings of awe and connection experienced while looking at a majestic mountain scene, or a beautiful sunset; gazing on a phenomenal work of art, or listening to a rapturous piece of music bringing tears to our eyes, as they serve as spectacular sources of creative inspiration. Sudden illumination, problem solving and creative insights are frequent occurrences when we allow ourselves to lapse into ASCs, be they induced trance, sleep, meditation, or even intoxication. I have known several people who claim that they received tremendous insights whilst inebriated, and these insights have been truly helpful in their lives.

ASCs in Social Situations.

This in and of itself is a huge subject; suffice to say I will touch on only a few areas here. When ASCs occur in a group setting they seem to serve both the individual, and the group, and can be seen as an integral part of many cultures.

Spirit possession provides us with an example of the benefits of social ASCs, as its impact and ramifications are considerable. In many indigenous cultures for example the local medicine man or shaman will often call in the spirits to possess him or her to create a healing. This ability gives the shaman his status amongst his people. Similar situations are said to occur in the western world when the Holy Spirit, Jesus or Mary possesses a religious leader or member of the congregation. Such possessions will often allow the possessed person to attain high status within his community, and allows a temporary freedom from his actions and proclamations. This can often be an excuse to act out in a socially acceptable way any aggressive, or even sexual conflicts and desires. The result is a dissipation of tensions and fears, and a new sense of spiritual connection and confidence may emerge.

From the community's perspective the group's needs are met through their vicarious association with the possessed person who is acting on behalf of the group as a whole. The possessed person will often derive personal satisfaction from the spiritual possession. He will often act out through ritual group conflicts and aspirations, such as death, resurrection and cultural taboos. The somewhat dramatic behaviours of the person possessed act as a reminder of the continued personal interest of their gods and reaffirms their cultural beliefs, while allowing them to have some perceived control over the unknown. It also provides an opportunity for group cohesion and reaffirms their identity, placing an importance on the utterances of the possessed person that they may not attain in a more ordinary setting. According to a number of researchers, the existence of such practices provides us with an example of how a society will naturally create ways of reducing frustration, stress and loneliness through group action.

The current research of many neuroscientists is enabling the general population to begin to understand without the need to fully believe that both the physiological and the psychological knowledge we collectively possess has value. It is highly liberating to realize that we do not need to take a specific stance to be able to explore our states of consciousness with a flexible and clear mind. This offers many people the opportunity to enjoy this exploration, and what they may discover.

Chapter III

A Personal Journey into Healing with ASCs

An uninvestigated life is not worth living.
(Socrates)

The non-attributed quotation, 'Life is a journey, not a destination' is a phrase often used in New Age literature. On hearing this, the questions that arise for me are, 'What does this actually mean? And, how does it apply to my work and research into ASCs and healing?' Fundamentally, the statement describes to me the foundation of this work as each day, each week, each month, something new is revealed to me. There is so much that remains unknown, and this work is a small step in revealing the power of our minds, along with our own innate abilities to heal.

As I stated in my introduction I started this journey of research and experiential learning as a strong sceptic, and yet now I find myself in a very different place. I have discovered many things about myself and the people with whom I work, and this enables me, and them to lead far healthier and fulfilling lives. In this section I will share with you my journey to date, and the role ASCs have played in moving me towards health and well-being.

Neuro Linguistic Programming
My very first experiences with ASCs came in the form of NLP (Neuro Linguistic Programming). I was a young chief executive in the health service, and was asked if I would pilot something called executive coaching. The purpose of this was to see how it could benefit other young women, who had aspirations to become senior executives. At that time, despite my rapid career progression I had not undertaken any personal development or training, other than my initial clinical degree. I therefore

embarked on my coaching with an expectation that this would simply be an interesting intellectual exercise.

How wrong could I have been? I went along to my first session with my selected coach, and what transpired left me feeling deeply uncomfortable. I was asked to explore parts of myself that I had never even considered before, and to participate in some rather strange (to my mind at the time) processes. These were my first experiences of ASCs. The results were quite amazing; after a few sessions, I found that I was feeling less stressed, and more in control of my life. It all still felt a bit strange, but I felt that I could trust my coach, and I genuinely began to enjoy the work I did with her. One day I asked her what she was 'doing to me?' She quite wisely told me that she was doing nothing 'to' me, but was simply enabling me to identify and create new options and possibilities for myself. I was intrigued, and enquired about how I could learn these skills to assist myself and others. There began my journey into working with and understanding ASCs.

In 1995 I trained to be an NLP practitioner with the intention of using my new skills in my exacting job as a health service executive. The training was quite a challenge for me. I discovered that I was very good at learning the processes and using these with my fellow students, however, I found that I was unable to fully allow other people to use the processes to full effect with me. Looking back, I see that I was unable to relax and let the processes unfold. I held on to a fear of letting go and allowing. At the end of each day, the trainer would guide us through a visualisation process which, I found profoundly unnerving. I would sit there with my eyes closed, mentally refusing to relax and follow his suggestions. I was terrified, literally scared stiff of letting go.

I was so firmly fixed within a left brain logical view of life that anything that was outside of this 'map of the world' was weird and frightening. With hindsight, I realise that I was so dissociated from my feelings, that I was unable to experience many of the beautiful and fulfilling aspects of life. However, at the time I was completely unaware of this. All I knew about then was using my brain to focus combined with a determination to succeed in my career. I qualified as an NLP practitioner with a very strong grasp of the mental processes of NLP without having learned much about working with my unconscious mind effectively.

But, my first tentative steps into the unknown had been taken. I left with one very clear outcome; I wanted to leave the health service to set up my own business. The reason for this was that I knew that with my newly acquired skills I had the abilities to help change the health care system for the better and, more specifically to assist the people within it. However, in order to do this I needed to leave the constraints of direct employment, and act as an external resource. Hence I returned to work following the end of my NLP Practitioner training and submitted my resignation. I knew deep inside of me, at a profound unconscious level that this was what I needed to do. This was a huge step for me, and it demonstrated that I was truly beginning to move beyond the constraints of my limited conscious awareness into the wider 'unknown.'

Hypnosis

During my NLP training a number of people had been talking about hypnosis. Initially, I had dismissed this as fantasy, but something clearly resonated inside of me as I began to hear about the positive experiences other people had with hypnosis. My curiosity was piqued, and I eventually found a 5-day hypnosis programme in London, which looked as if it would offer me an introduction to hypnosis. My conscious intention was that this programme would enable me to 'test out hypnosis to prove that it wouldn't work on me.' I had never thought of myself as an arrogant person, but on reflection, my assumptions about hypnosis were tinged with what can only be called arrogance.

Hence, it was in this frame of mind that I attended the training. Here I encountered another key turning point in my thinking and way of being.

The trainer was Tad James, who I now consider as one of the best hypnotherapy technicians in the world. His use of language was precise and exquisite. I sat back in my usual dissociated state and 'observed'. Despite my learnings on my NLP Practitioner training, I was still a long way from allowing things to unfold. I watched as Tad demonstrated the various techniques, and I participated to a limited degree, as much as I felt able, in the group exercises.

At one point during the first day, something shifted fundamentally within me; I had the realisation that I was totally in control! I could choose to do as suggested by the hypnotherapist or not, I could stop the process at any time that I chose. I started to laugh. This was the kind of deep, gurgling laugh that comes when we are faced with a truism that suddenly hits us as so obvious that we can't believe that we hadn't seen it before. It is as if the childlike attitude of my unconscious mind had finally broken through the constraints of my very serious and adult conscious mind.

This was a huge turning point for me, a true life-changing event. In that moment I decided that I needed to understand myself more, to understand the roots of the fear that had brought me to this moment, and to start to explore the aspects of my mind that were other than conscious. The journey had truly begun. After the course ended, I began to meet up with one of the people I had met on the course to practise the techniques we had been taught. A whole new world began to unfold for me. I found that the more I went into trance, the easier it became, and the deeper I could go. I began to be fascinated by the changes I was able to make in my life simply by tapping into different levels of consciousness. My rampant blood pressure came in to alignment, my weight rebalanced, and I began to feel I had a lot more energy and enthusiasm for life. I realised that prior to this moment I had forgotten what it was like to enjoy life and feel fulfilled. My work was rewarding, I had started a consultancy practice, and yet I knew with my new deepening awareness of myself that something within this needed to change, and hypnosis provided me with the tools to do this.

I had also begun a practice of meditation; another way of accessing ASCs. I found that spending twenty minutes in the morning in meditation enabled me to feel balanced and relaxed as I went about my daily activities. On the occasional times when I was unable to do this, I quickly noticed that I felt really different, and my days did not go so smoothly. Lowering my brainwave activity at least once a day through meditation, self hypnosis, or using a guided visualisation CD soon became a very important and integral part of my day.

Advanced NLP and Much More

After attending the 5-day hypnosis course in London I decided to attend Tad James' NLP Master Practitioner training in Hawaii. The course offered qualifications in hypnosis and Time Line Therapy ™ as well as NLP, which I felt would offer me a broader experience. This training once again provided me with other experiences that opened me up to the potential of ASCs. I found that during the training I had the opportunity to face many of my demons. I had nowhere to hide; I was the only person from the UK with the majority of the class being from the USA and Canada. The energy of the islands also had a huge impact on me. This combined with the fact that I was in and out of ASCs during the course everyday facilitated fundamental changes within me. I began to challenge my hitherto limited views of the world and my role within it.

With the help and patience of my classmates, I was able to clear away a huge number of blockages to experiencing a loving and fulfilling life. I was able to allow myself to go into full body catalepsy, which was a profoundly healing experience. I was fully aware of the people around me, and even knew that someone had taken a photograph. I didn't know who had taken the photo until it arrived in the mail several months later. In this state I had reached a very deep level of ASC where a truly profound healing had taken place. I felt renewed, energised, and whole for the first time in my adult life.

The healing power of the Hawaiian Islands also introduced me to the ability to tune in to, and work with nature spirits and the spirits of the earth, sky and ocean by entering into ASCs. I could feel something very special on the islands which I had never felt before. I would spend as much time as I could sitting alone in the He'au's surrounding the hotel, and allow myself to connect with the spirit energies; I would swim in the ocean, and meditate each morning floating in the warm ocean. Each morning I would get up and go down to the beach, and every time two or three turtles would join me as I swam and meditated.

One morning the ocean was very choppy, but as I am a strong swimmer I decided to proceed with my morning practice. The waves were strong, and at one point I found myself being thrown towards the sharp coral by a huge wave. Just before I was about to hit the sharp coral one of my turtle friends positioned himself between me and the jagged coral so that I floated safely past the potential danger. On another occasion I was visiting the sacred Place of Refuge on the Big Island, and went to meditate on a peninsula by the ocean's edge. When I opened my eyes I was surrounded by turtles floating in the water, their little heads bobbing up and down. Many indigenous cultures talk about people having specific totem animals who work with us to bring balance and healing. One of my totem animals is certainly the turtle.

I knew at this point in time that a deep level of healing was only possible by allowing me to enter into deeper ASCs. I also knew that I needed to be able to teach others to do this, so that they too could receive the healing benefits. Ever since that time, I have not experienced any of the grumbling illnesses that I used to get such as irritable bowel, chronic stomach problems, recurrent influenza, and 'Monday morning 5 a.m. sickness.' I come from a family who is constantly getting bugs and illnesses, and as a child I had all of the childhood diseases several times, including those that medical science said were only possible to have once. So my medical history was quite interesting. I am now fit and in robust health whereas the rest of my family have chosen to remain in the cycle of dis-ease.

About eight months later, I attended Tad's Trainers training programme. Here every obstacle that was in my path seemed to be blown away and I found myself on yet another new track in my life. During the programme I booked a massage to assist me in physically integrating the mental-emotional changes I was making in my life. During the massage I entered into a deep ASC when I became aware that I was floating above the massage table. My physical body had levitated off the table and my therapist was holding onto my ankles saying, 'It is OK, I won't let go!' I had lifted about eight inches off the massage table and remained there for what seemed like a very long time. However, it was probably only seconds before my conscious mind kicked back in, and I was lying back on the massage table. I was exhausted and exhilarated both at the same time. It was as if I had entered into an ASC so deep that gravity no longer affected my physical body in the usual way. After this experience my body quickly released the excess weight I had begun to re-accumulate, and I felt renewed once more. This experience along with several others at around the same time in my life caused me to want to explore more deeply the possibilities of ASCs in healing and returning to wholeness.

As I had more and more positive experiences with ASCs I noticed that the work I was doing with my clients was also changing. When I started my consultancy business in early

1996, I was predominately undertaking analytical projects, writing strategic documents, and making recommendations for organisational change. As my own consciousness shifted I noticed that I was attracting different clients, and my work was becoming more individually based. This was wrapped in the disguise of coaching, which over time began to be more akin to pure therapy sessions. It was as if every time I took a step forward in my own development, and use of ASCs in their various guises, I attracted new clients who required similar work themselves. This had the effect of clarifying my own learning, whilst enabling others to benefit from this simultaneously.

Whilst at my NLP trainers training I met, and subsequently married, my current partner. He and I have grown together and challenged each other on every level during the eleven years of our relationship. Thankfully, we have similar interests, and have therefore been able to attend a number of trainings together.

Fire Walking

As my confidence of working with and using ASCs grew, I began to explore past life regression therapy, fire walking, and plant medicine, as well as bending construction reinforcement bars and breaking arrows with my throat. I was continually pushing at the boundaries of my understanding of myself and life. Another of my quantum leaps was made when I found myself being drawn to the notion of fire walking. I ultimately found an experienced instructor and learned how to fire walk, and in due course became a fire walk instructor. There was no logical reason for me to want to do this other than to push the boundaries of my current learning and understanding. However, I felt a really strong desire to learn about the benefits of walking on fire. I had seen and indeed experienced some of what I call the macho approach to fire walking. I felt that there was something fundamentally missing from this approach, which seemed to be about 'conquering' rather than 'working with' the fire. Finally, I found a programme which was being run by Peggy Dylan, who is one of the people responsible for bringing fire walking into the awareness of the western world in the 1980s and 1990s.

One of the key learnings that I had during my apprenticeship to become a fire walk instructor was once more about using energy to enter into an ASC. The fundamental tenet of successful fire walking is that when our energy matches the energy of the fire we can walk safely. I was trained to connect with the energy of the fire by entering into an ASC. In this place we can then develop a kind of symbiotic relationship with the fire enabling us to understand when it is safe to walk on the hot coals. People will often ask me how they will know when it is safe to walk. My reply is that they will 'simply know'. Something inside tells us when it is safe to walk and hearing that voice is only possible when we are in an ASC. I know that when I approached the fire for the first time I could feel that I was in a distinctly altered state, my heart was pumping and my knees felt weak, and yet I knew it was the time to walk. When I stepped off the coals at the other end of the walk I felt absolutely complete and elated. The thought that came to me was, 'If you can do that, what can't you do?' If we can do the seemingly impossible, what is truly impossible? I do not yet know the answer to this, but the more I explore ASCs and their potential for human consciousness, the more I am convinced that we know very little about our true potential.

The most powerful experience I have ever had with fire walking and healing was once again during my fire walk instructor apprenticeship. One evening we built a fire together as a group, and then returned to the lodge where we were staying. Each one of us in turn went down to the fire, raked it out and walked on it alone, raking the coals back into a pile for the next person. I found this to be a profoundly emotional experience. I sat with the fire, and set my intentions to connect with its essence to enable me to walk safely. I also wanted to heal a small patch of chronic eczema. I found myself overcome by emotion; I slipped into an ASC which felt so beautiful that tears rolled down my cheeks. I had a profound feeling of wholeness and oneness with the fire and the earth. I reverently raked out the coals, walked across them. Then I very carefully piled the coals up for the next person. I returned to the lodge in a deeply peaceful state of mind, feeling like a very different person. I then looked at the sole of my foot where the eczema had been, and it was gone.

Another important lesson I learned about ASCs, healing and energy during my fire walk instructor apprenticeship was about the alignment of group energy. We were divided (and I use this word advisedly) into three groups to manage the various aspects of a fire walk evening. One group was tasked to build the fire, one to tend, and one to manage the actual walk. I was placed in the group to manage the walk itself. We had quite a discussion in the group about how we were going to manage our part of the walk. There were several opposing ideas and quite a lot of disagreement as egos kicked in to play. When it was time to walk we went to the fire site, and I instantly felt something was badly wrong. It felt like energies were pulling in different directions and I was finding it difficult to get myself into the ASC required to hold the energy and space needed for a safe and successful walk. One of my colleagues and I attempted to smooth the energy, but I found it really difficult to stay in any form of ASC. I realized the potential danger, and decided to stop the walk. I knew inherently that if anyone walked they would be hurt. Despite our warnings and concerns, one person still chose to walk, and this resulted in them receiving quite a nasty burn. The lesson I learned from this is: that in order for the healing of the fire to work, a group needs to be working together; egos need to be put aside, and the whole group in harmony. This enables the participants to enter into an ASC to walk safely and enable healing to occur.

Plant Medicine

The use of hallucinogenic and recreational drugs to 'escape' has always been something I steered clear of during my university years and beyond. However, in the last few years I had begun to become interested in working with plants in a more spiritual way, and read a lot about the use of Teacher Plants in indigenous cultures. My research led me to the conclusion that maybe there was some benefit in working with these plants as an avenue into holistic healing. Therefore, in the spring of 2008 I arranged to go to Peru with a small group of people to experience the sacred ceremonies of San Pedro and Ayahuasca.

Connecting with the spirits of the plants and working with them once again proved to be a watershed for me. We travelled to the foothills of the Andes where we experienced two beautiful San Pedro ceremonies, which lasted well into the night. The first was a cleansing ceremony where we drank the San Pedro liquid, and went through various rituals in order to purify ourselves on all levels. This involved quite a considerable amount of physical purging. I found myself entering into an ASC about twenty minutes after taking the bitter liquid. The whole ceremony was very beautiful and lasted well into the night, at the end I went to bed feeling very serene and at peace. The second ceremony scheduled two days later was nothing short of phenomenal. If I hadn't personally had the experience I would not have believed that it had happened.

The ceremony started at about ten in the evening, the sky was jet black, and I remember thinking that the sky seemed to be vibrating with glistening stars. One by one we drank the acrid juice and sat in a circle as the shaman began his work. We were each called in turn to stand in front of him to enable him to conduct his healings with each one of us.

When it was my turn, I stood about ten feet away from the Maestro (shaman) in the pitch dark. He was very still for the longest time, quietly chanting an icaro (sacred song). During this time I felt my grip on consensual reality loosen, as I entered into a profoundly altered state. I also felt a strong pull in the area of my power chakra (sternum). He suddenly mentioned my husband, Robert, saying that he thought that he was very sick and in severe danger. He said that it felt like Robert was suffering from something like a Santeria type 'curse', and then the shaman started to vomit. He told me that my husband had become very ill in the last twelve months, and also that he was wasting a lot of money and energy. I was shocked to the core as no one knew that my husband had been drinking very heavily, and had taken steps to end his life just months before. He also told me that Robert used to help people and that he could no longer do this. Again a profound truth; Robert had been a very successful therapist up until two years ago when he quite suddenly become depressed and unable to function effectively let alone work. He had continued to refuse any help which was a source of great sadness to me.

The shaman then asked me to focus my thoughts on Robert, and to close my eyes. I stood in front of him with my eyes closed, and felt myself enter into an even deeper ASC. I felt as if I was swaying, as if I was being 'pulled' backwards and forwards by some invisible force, and yet I felt like I was unable to move with any volition. I also felt a flood of tears rolling down my face. It was as if I was no longer fully present, that part of me had entered into a completely different reality, and yet at the same time I felt physically nauseas. I suddenly felt myself relax and allow the process to unfold. The shaman continued with his work, singing icaros and chanting. After some time he asked me how I felt, and I told him the nausea had passed. He sang a final icaro and camayed (sprayed) me with aqua florida, a sacred water. I finally returned to my place in the circle, completely exhausted. The next day one of my companions told me I had stood in front of the shaman for over 2 hours, and that he had seen a tube of vibrating light connecting me to the shaman throughout that time.

When I flew to Iquitos a few days later I phoned my husband. He told me that one morning he had awoken very early, and found he had more energy than he had had for a long time. He felt as if he wanted to do things and get on with life. I asked him which morning this was, and was intrigued to discover that it coincided exactly with the night I had undertaken my work with the shaman. The shaman working with the San Pedro plant had used me as a conduit to work with my sick husband. Both the shaman and I had entered into a collaborative, deep ASC in order for him to do this amazing work. Now, six months later Robert is enjoying life, and starting a new career as a rare breeds' farmer. I still look back on that experience with a great deal of incredulousness as there was nothing my logical mind could latch on to, however, what I do know is that it has worked. This occurred without my husband even consciously knowing anything was transpiring all those thousands of miles away across the Atlantic Ocean.

I remained in a deep sense of awe as we travelled into the Amazon to work with an Ayahuascero (a shaman who works with the ayahuasca vine, known as the Teacher Plant to the local people). Once again the ayahuasca ceremonies started in the evening around nine o'clock when the jungle was alive with its nightly chorus. On the first evening I felt anxious as I stepped into the communal lodge to start the first ceremony. I had read a lot about plant medicine and the effects this plant, Mother Ayahuasca, the great teacher plant, had on people. However my purpose in being there was to heal my blood pressure which had once again started to rise, and to heal myself from the effects of my husband's depression. When the ceremony started we took it in turns to stand, say a brief prayer, and quickly down the medicine. The taste was so acrid that it was very hard to swallow. I gulped it down quickly, and immediately began to feel nauseas. Thankfully, I managed to stay in my seat to allow the medicine to do its work. I felt the ayahuasca heating my stomach and radiating throughout my body as I began to enter into an ASC. Many of the other people vomited profusely, but for me it felt as if the brew needed to remain inside my stomach in order to work.

During the time I spent in the Amazon working with the Mother plant, I received a number of visions, and when I slept I had very vivid dreams. It was as if the ceremonies continued in my dream time. I spent a week purging my physical body and receiving these visions. The most powerful insight I had was when I realized that many of the visions I was receiving during the ceremonies, and the pictures the shaman drew, were actually of DNA. I was shown the strands of DNA and the minute workings of our bodies. This was the clue I needed to understand how the shamans do their healing. They use plant medicine to enter into an ASC which enables them to see what is required to heal on a cellular level. I was bowled over by this realization. This was later confirmed for me by the Swiss anthropologist Jeremy Narby in his book, *The Cosmic Serpent,* (1999).

Chapter IV

Hypnotic Processes

Hypnosis

Lewis Wolfberg (2007) suggests that the earliest legitimate recorded description of hypnosis can be found in Genesis 2.21-21.

And the Lord God caused a deep sleep to fall upon Adam, and he slept, and he took one of his ribs, and closed up the flesh instead thereof. And the rib, which the Lord God had taken from man, made he a woman, and brought her unto the man.

Other texts suggest that hypnosis dates back around three thousand years or more in the Egyptian sleep temples. Little is written about this, however, based on my own research into indigenous cultures I would suggest that this was more likely to be some other form of ASC rather than the type of hypnosis that we know today.

Mesmer is probably one of the better known early proponents of hypnosis. According to the history of hypnosis, it is said that (*James*, 1996) in 1776 Franz Mesmer created the dawn of clinical hypnosis. He described that cosmic and planetary magnetism could be contained in bodies of people, and animals (animal magnetism). He also stated that it could be 'transmitted' by magnetic passes, and that people differ in their abilities to transfer magnetism. However, a commission of nine eminent scientists, including Benjamin Franklin, said there was nothing to his theories, and Mesmer was ultimately discredited.

In 1850, James Esdaile, a Scottish surgeon during the wars in India, performed over a thousand surgical operations using hypnosis. However, it was not until 1955 that the BMA, (The British Medical Association) acknowledged hypnosis as an acceptable and legitimate medical procedure. The AMA (American Medical Association) followed suit three years later.

Hypnosis is currently used successfully to assist people in a wide range of situations from building self-confidence and stopping smoking, through to creating profound healings, such as recovery from cancers, and other life-threatening diseases.

According to the World Heath Organization (WHO), (2008) ninety per cent of the world's general population are capable of being hypnotised. Despite the popular notion that hypnosis is something extra-ordinary, it is a naturally occurring ASC, which we experience on a daily basis. Most people enter into this natural state several times a day when they are deeply engrossed in a book, a movie, or driving along the highway and do not recall the journey. When we are deeply focused on something, and do not hear someone talking to us we are in an ASC or hypnotic trance.

The hypnotic state is very helpful in that it produces a profound state of relaxation. However, the real power of hypnosis is that in this relaxed state we are able to open our minds, and become receptive to suggestions, which can result in healing (*Yarnell*, 2008). This state enables positive and healing suggestions to sink in much more quickly and deeply than when we are in an 'up-time' alert state. I have been asked by numerous people why it is that only positive suggestions are accepted by the unconscious mind while people are in a hypnotic state. During my extensive research into the subject, I have not found a single example of how hypnosis has been used to suggest that someone do something that they would not normally do. It seems that our unconscious mind has a sense of morality, and hence will reject suggestions that are outside of its own moral code (*James*, 1996).

Personal Practice

Often when a client comes to me for hypnosis for the first time, they tend to have tried several other routes to resolve their issue or illness. Having been down these routes, they are ready to try something different. They are often apprehensive and nervous, usually because they have heard many stories about hypnosis. I therefore take time to get to know the person and what makes them tick, along with their medical history and any 'treatments' they may have already had. This not only gives me insight into their story but it also enables me to develop a deep level of rapport. Once I have this degree of rapport, I ask them about any concerns they may have about hypnosis, and take the time to allay any of their fears and misconceptions.

I usually say something like the following; 'I don't know about you, but I like to think I am in control of myself and any given situation. You know, the reason I went on my first hypnosis course was to prove to myself that it did not work! I had learned NLP, and a lot of people on my course were talking about hypnosis. I was very sceptical, and yet curious. I therefore decided to go on a course to learn more about hypnosis. I ultimately attended a five-day programme, and was amazed at what I discovered. First, I found that it was great fun, and importantly I discovered that I was in control of the whole process when I was "being the client". The truly amazing thing about hypnosis I discovered was that the client, not the hypnotherapist, is in control. The client is ultimately at choice about whether they follow the suggestions of the hypnotherapist. Once I had proved this I was very happy, and I took further training to qualify as a clinical hypnotherapist.'

The following is an example of how I will often discuss hypnosis with a new client. The language used here is not grammatically correct as it is used to create a trance state, and bypasses the client's unconscious mind, going directly to their unconscious mind.

'When you and I work together, I want you to know that only you can make the decision to follow what I say, or not. I can guide you into a relaxed hypnotic state, where you can choose to follow my suggestions or not, it is up to you. Hypnosis has been used for several centuries to assist people in healing themselves and alleviating problems. During our time together, you will do your own healing; my role is simply to guide you to where you can heal this situation for yourself. Hypnosis enables you to connect with that part of yourself that can heal you, the part that contains the blueprint of perfect health.

'I have worked with a lot of people, including myself to bring balance and health into their lives. People have overcome life-threatening dis-eases such as cancer, and quit antisocial habits such as smoking and nail biting. Hypnosis is a non-dependent healing process that enables you to heal yourself without any drugs or chemicals; it is a completely natural process. It can also help to make allopathic treatments more effective. Are you ready to proceed or do you have any questions?'

I would then answer any questions the client has and then proceed with a relaxing induction and hypnotic session.

N.B. If the client is taking medications, or is having any other type of medical treatment, I will contact the client's doctor, in order that we can work together to assist our client/patient in healing.

As a hypnotherapist, the hypnotic inductions I use to guide my clients into ASCs simply focus their attention in order that they can move naturally into a hypnotic trance state. Some hypnotherapists believe that repetition is important to enable change, and therefore repeated sessions are required to enable someone to heal fully. However, I have worked with numerous clients, and on most occasions they only need one or two sessions before their problems completely disappear. I therefore think that the beliefs of the therapist are a fundamental part of their client's healing process. I have recently worked with a client whose mother is a therapist. The young woman came to see me, and the first words she said were, 'I know that this is going to take a long time to sort out.' Hence the first thing I had to do was help her to release this negative belief in order to resolve the issue for which she came to consult me.

During the course of my practice, it has become evident that it is important for all hypnotic change to be self-generated. I therefore choose not to work with people who want to come to see me for smoking cessation, for example, if their husband or wife wants them to quit. This is because these people may not truly wish to change at a deep level, but are coming for the sessions to appease their partner. This attitude has the effect of reducing the success of the work. I will usually say to these people, 'Come back and see me when *you* are really ready to change.'

The other aspect of this work that I have found to be of paramount importance is to ensure that any suggestions made are plausible within my client's belief system. This enables their unconscious mind to accept the suggestions easily. As a hypnotherapist it is therefore important to elicit a client's beliefs and values at the outset of a session to ensure that any suggestions given will be readily accepted by the client's unconscious mind. In fact, on occasion if I am using a direct authoritarian style (see below) of hypnosis, I will ask the client directly what suggestions they would like me to make. This ensures I am using their words, which are immediately recognizable by their unconscious mind.

Demystifying Hypnosis

Hypnosis is often made to seem mysterious or complicated, and yet it is a simple process, which can also be elegant and enjoyable. Words act as triggers, enabling us to create pictures in our mind. A good example of this is when we read a novel; we create our own movie as we read the book. I have observed that quite often when someone has read a book, and a movie is then made based on the book, people will often say, 'It was ok, but it wasn't as good as the book.' This is because we have a great imagination; we create pictures that appeal to us, which are more often than not quite different from someone else's.

Some people create the pictures in their mind quickly, while other people need a little more time. This is because each individual processes information, and creates images in their minds, based on their preferred representational systems. In his book, *Hypnosis for Beginners*, Dylan Morgan (2003) states the following:

- Words trigger pictures in the mind
- It takes a little time for us to create these pictures
- The time this takes varies from person to person

When we use our imagination to create pictures we are entering into an ASC. A hypnotherapist uses this ability to induce these states, and elicit change. All change occurs at the unconscious level, and so hypnosis enables us to open a doorway to our unconscious mind where the desired change can occur.

According to Lesley LeCron, here are six different levels, or depths of trance that can be induced through hypnosis (1964).

Level one
Lethargy
Relaxation | Light Level trance |
Eye catalepsy

Level two
Catalepsy of isolated muscle groups | Light Level trance |
Heavy or floating feelings

Level three
Rapport
Smell and taste changes
Number block

Level four

Amnesia

Analgesia

Automatic movement

Medium Level trance

Level five

Positive auditory and visual hallucinations

Bizarre post hypnotic suggestions

Level six

Negative hallucinations

Comatose

Somnambulism

Deep Level trance

While it can be helpful in discussing levels of trance with clients, these various depths of hypnosis are ostensibly arbitrary delineations as no two people respond to hypnosis in an identical or even similar manner. Depth can also vary within the same person dependent upon their mental-emotional state at the time of trance induction. Over time, I have personally experienced that going into trance is easier, and I can attain deeper levels, than when I first started to learn and use hypnosis. However, there are times when my conscious mind is very active and I find it more difficult to go into trance.

The purpose of defining the three major levels of trance is listed as follows:

Light level hypnosis – The single most important aspect in achieving any level of hypnotic trance is to first facilitate the client in accepting the validity of simple suggestions, and then to build up into suggestions that are more complex.

Medium level hypnosis – Limb catalepsy followed by the suggestion of deep relaxation furthers belief. As the level of trance deepens, the sub cortical areas of the brain take over as in the sleep state.

Somnambulism or deep level hypnosis – conviction at this level is complete and there is no need for reality testing. The hypnotherapist's suggestions are received literally without any intervention by the client's conscious mind. Hence, the suggestions given cannot be compared with previous data, so they are accepted fully as convictions. If it is not present, amnesia can be produced by a simple suggestion.

Both positive and negative hallucinations are produced easily because the person's beliefs grow with conviction. This often results in an increase in voluntary performance.

Approaches to Hypnosis

Modern day hypnotherapists tend to use one, and or both, of the two popular types of induction. The first is called the *Direct Authoritarian approach,* which appeals directly to the client's conscious mind. The down side to this approach is that it can provide the client with the opportunity to evaluate the procedure as their conscious mind is engaged in the process. The purpose is to direct the client through a series of instructions, fixing attention on the hypnotherapist's voice. The second approach is the *Indirect Permissive approach,* where indirect suggestions bypass the conscious mind, going directly to the unconscious mind. For example:

Direct approach, 'Close the door.'

Indirect approach, 'I am wondering if you can, close the door.'

There are many scripts available for use in the direct approach whereas the indirect approach relies more upon the hypnotherapist utilizing naturally occurring physiological functions and external stimuli. George Estabrooks and Dave Elman were two of the great masters of direct authoritarian hypnosis, whereas, Milton Erickson was the master and largely the creator of the indirect approach. I have personally found that using a combination of the two styles can be very powerful for people who have a very active conscious mind. The direct approach serves to occupy their conscious mind, whilst simultaneously working with their unconscious mind.

Probably the best way to describe these two different approaches to hypnotic induction is to provide examples of both.

Direct Authoritarian Induction (Elman)

Stage 1 – eye lid closure

'Now take a long deep breath and hold it for a few seconds.

'As you exhale this breath, allow your eyelids to close, and let go of the surface tension in your body. Just let your body relax as much as possible right now.' *(Eye closure.)*

'Now, place your awareness on your eye muscles and relax the muscles around your eyes to the point that they just won't work. When you are sure that they are so relaxed that as long as you hold onto this relaxation, they just won't work, hold on to that relaxation and test them, to make sure THEY WON'T WORK.' *(Eye catalepsy.)*

Stage two – physical relaxation

'Now this relaxation you have in your eyes is the same quality of relaxation I want you to have throughout your whole body. So, just let this quality of relaxation flow through your whole body from the top of your head, to the tips of your toes.' *(Relaxation spreading through the body.)*

'Now we can deepen this relaxation much more. In a moment, I am going to have you open and close your eyes, double the relaxation you now have. Make it twice as deep. Ok, now, once more open your eyes... close your eyes and double your relaxation... good. Let every muscle in your body become so relaxed that as long as you hold onto this quality of relaxation, every muscle of your body will not work.'

Stage three – somnambulism

'In a moment, I'll ask you to begin slowly counting backward, out loud, from 100. Now, here's the secret to mental relaxation, with each number you say, double your mental relaxation. With each number you say, let your mind become twice as relaxed.' (*Mental relaxation.*)

'Now by the time you reach the number 98, or maybe even sooner, your mind will have become so relaxed, you will have actually relaxed all the rest of the numbers that would have come after 98 right out of your mind, there just won't be any more numbers. Now, you have to do this, I cannot do it for you. Those numbers will leave if you will them away. Now start with the idea that you will make that happen and you can easily dispel them from your mind. Want it to happen, will it to happen, make it happen.' (*Number block.*)

'Double your mental relaxation. Start to make those numbers leave. They'll go if you will them away.'

'Now they'll be gone. Dispel them. Banish them. Make it happen, you can do it; I can't do it for you. Put them out. Make it happen! ARE THEY ALL GONE?'(*Amnesia.*)

Stage four – coma (also known as the Esdaile state)

'The closest I can come to describing mental relaxation is to have you think of yourself as an infant before you fall asleep. Shortly before sleep actually comes, the mind becomes a complete blank, and then you drift off to sleep. In my opinion, when the mind is almost completely inactive, mental relaxation is achieved.'(*Totally 'out'.*)

The above induction specifically instructs the client through the various stages described and used by Dave Elman (1964). Explicit directions are given for the client to follow. This is in contrast to the indirect approach described below which asks a series of questions to elicit trance.

Indirect Ericksonian approach

An example of this more permissive approach to inductions (*James, 1996*) is as follows:

'Have you ever been in a trance before... right now?'

If the answer to this question is, no, then ask a supplementary question, 'What is the relationship between the state you are in right now and the state you were in just before you woke this morning?'

'Did you experience the hypnotic state as basically similar to the waking state or different?'

'Would you like to find a spot above eye level that (looking up helps to bring on an alpha level ASC) you can look at comfortably?'

'As you continue looking at that spot for a while, do your eyelids want to blink?'

'Will those lids begin to blink together or separately?'

'Slowly or quickly?'

'Will they close all at once or flutter by themselves first?'

'Will those eyes close more and more as you get more and more comfortable?'

'That's fine. Can those eyes now remain closed as your comfort deepened, like when you go to sleep?'

'Can that comfort continue more and more so that you'd rather not even try to open your eyes?'

'Or would you rather try and find that you cannot?'

'And how quickly will you forget about them all together because (pause) your unconscious wants to dream?'

Suggestions can then be inserted in here before bringing the client out of trance as follows:

'In a moment I am going to count backwards from 10 to 1, and I want you to awaken 1/10th of the way with each number until you are fully awake. 10... 9... 8...'

Counting can be done backwards as in this example or forwards from 1 up to 10 to achieve full awareness, whichever is the preferred style of the hypnotherapist.

As can be seen, the above induction allows the client to search for answers to the questions and the act of searching itself sends them into a trance. With each subsequent question, they go deeper into trance. Each question offers a perceived choice, which enables the client to feel as if they are fully in control. Some hypnotherapists use a combination of indirect and direct inductions very effectively. However, I personally find that I can use the Ericksonian indirect approach alone with almost every client to great effect.

The diagram below is taken from my original Master Hypnosis Training manual (*James, 1996*).

Multiple Embedded Metaphors

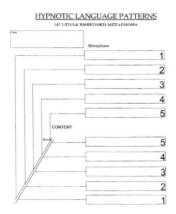

Figure 3: Multiple Embedded Metaphors

I have found the use of multiple embedded metaphors to be invaluable when working with clients either on an individual basis or in groups. The process is quite simple; first, if I am running a training programme I will usually wish to elicit a particular mental-emotional state such as curiosity or excitement about learning something new. I then identify about five metaphors that will assist me in eliciting these states in the group. Once I have these metaphors, I enter into the state of curiosity or excitement, and begin to tell the first story until I am about 75 per cent of the way through. I then slip seamlessly into the second metaphor, and tell 75 per cent of that, repeating the process with all five metaphors. I then deliver the message I wish to impart, and then I tell the remaining 25 per cent of the metaphors in reverse order staring with the fifth, and finishing with the first. The sense of curiosity elicited alters the group's state of consciousness, and they become more open and curious, enabling them to pay more attention to the messages I am giving. The term used by Tad James when he initially taught me this process in 1996 was that this is like locking something into a Tupperware box. The message between the metaphors could be as short as a simple suggestion or as long as a whole training, several days long.

Components of Hypnosis

Suggestibility

Most people believe that it is the hypnotherapist who produces the responses to hypnotic suggestions; however it is actually the client who initiates the response based on previously experienced conditioning (*Kroger, 1973*). Misdirection can reduce criticalness, enabling a suggestion to be accepted unconditionally by passing the client's conscious mind. A person increases in their suggestibility with the more suggestions that are given. This is called abstract conditioning, and helps us to understand the role that suggestibility plays in the production of hypnotic phenomena.

Suggestibility is enhanced by the motivation of the client. Its effectiveness is principally dependant on the level of rapport between the hypnotist/hypnotherapist and the client. Suggestibility in itself does not account for hypnotisability; however, increased suggestibility is a constant feature of hypnosis. The research by Kroger suggests that suggestibility is slightly greater in females with a male hypnotist. However, it can also be argued that as suggestibility depends on motivation, it varies from person to person, including emotional changes in the same person. In my own experience, the prestige of the person making the suggestions in relation to the client is more likely to be a key influence. Kroger also states that someone may be highly suggestible to stimuli affecting his health, yet non suggestible to persuasive salesmanship. This is because his critical factors are aroused in the latter. Interestingly the same person could also be highly suggestible to religious suggestions if they fit with their value systems.

The level of suggestibility cannot be evaluated in advance. It is fascinating that paradoxical clients, who believe they are not suggestible, almost always react with positive suggestibility because of their innate stubbornness.

Catalepsy

Catalepsy is another aspect of hypnosis, which is characterised by a peculiar involuntary increase in the elastic tension of the muscles. Limbs will remain in almost any position in which they are placed. In eyeball catalepsy, the eyes do not move when the head is turned slowly, but remain fixed as the head is turned. Catalepsy usually denotes that a medium trance has been achieved. This is a good guide to enable the hypnotherapist to know the level of trance that they have achieved with their client.

I use catalepsy as an indicator when I am working with clients who respond well to direct authoritarian hypnosis for a range of healings. I have used it successfully with people who have angina and had a recent heart attack, asthma, diabetes, weight issues, cancer and arthritis.

Post hypnotic suggestions and conditioning

Post hypnotic phenomena are acts which are carried out following a hypnotic session in response to specific suggestions made by the hypnotherapist. The stimulus is the suggestion given during hypnosis, and the actions become the response. A post-hypnotic action is often a complex task completed as a result of a single 'learning' session. It is more durable than a conditioned reflex, and is less easily turned off.

A post hypnotic suggestion can last for minutes or years. According to Kroger, it is generally agreed that a suggestion will usually last up to two months. During this time it will weaken, however, periodic reinforcement tends to increase its effectiveness. Post hypnotic suggestions are generally followed no matter what the depth of trance. These suggestions should be in keeping with the client's values and beliefs to prevent unnecessary anxiety and internal conflict.

Some people will develop a complete conscious amnesia about the suggestions, and yet will readily follow them. Others will have full recall, and still follow them. Another group of people will recall the suggestion once the act has been completed. This is akin to compulsive behaviours, we know what we are doing, but we do not know why. If circumstances change significantly between the time of the suggestion, and when it is to be carried out, then the client can often cancel the original suggestion. It is as if we have a hard-wired intelligent safety mechanism.

If a post hypnotic suggestion is out of alignment with the client's desires, and it is still carried out, the client will usually rationalize this unusual behaviour. Part of our built in safeguard is that purposeless post hypnotic suggestions are as easily forgotten as similar instructions given in a non-hypnotic state.

Amnesia

Amnesia can spontaneously occur during a hypnotic session, it is however, more frequently produced with post hypnotic suggestions. Following hypnosis when amnesia has occurred, there is a selective loss of memory. The client is unaware of what transpired during the hypnotically induced amnesia, however, these memories are simply held in abeyance. When the client is re-hypnotised they will normally recall almost everything that happened during the previous session, others will gradually forget all, or some of their experiences.

Amnesia is actually an everyday experience; we can temporarily forget the name of a lifelong friend when we go to introduce them to someone. Spontaneous or suggested amnesia gives us an indication of the depth of the hypnotic trance, the latter is indicative of a deep level of trance known as somnambulism. An easy way to induce post hypnotic amnesia is to say something like, 'When you open your eyes, you will have no recollection of what I have said to you whilst you were in a trance. However, all of the suggestions I have given you will be carried out as I specified.'

Dissociation

Dissociation is the inherent ability of the hypnotised person to 'detach' themselves from the immediate environment. This can also happen in a non-hypnotised state, such as being in a reverie. The person can be completely dissociated and yet be able to function effectively. This state is similar to the lucid dreaming state, when a person can see himself or herself undertaking specific activities.

Someone who is well practised at hypnosis can often 'step out' of himself, and see himself sitting on the other side of the room. Dissociation can be used to induce hypnoanaesthesia. For example, a comment made to a deeply hypnotised patient sitting in a dental chair can increase their pain threshold, or a body part can be anaesthetised through dissociation, with the person not feeling the separated part.

Depersonalisation

Depersonalisation can be simply induced in a suggestible client with post hypnotic suggestions. Clients can be told to forget their own identity and assume that of another person. Depersonalisation is also used psychotherapeutically in a similar way to dissociation.

Revivification and age regression

Revivification and age regression are different from each other. Revivification is the reliving of earlier events through hypnosis when all the memories of life following those events are temporarily lost. Age regression differs in that the client plays a role, acting out past life events in the present day framework. This form of age regression is called pseudorevivification.

Revivification is produced by post hypnotic suggestions where the client exhibits many of the personality traits of that time in their lives. This can be seen as childlike words and handwriting. Misremembering can occur in response to prior suggestion that a specific thing took place. However, recall is greatly improved under hypnosis when strong emotional elements are associated with the memories.

Theories of Hypnosis

There are many different theories about hypnosis just as there are about human behaviour.

Listed below are a number of these *(Crasilneck & James, 1985):*

Atavistic hypothesis: immobilisation theories

Kroger and Freed (1973) suggested that hypnotic behaviour is an atavism that may have been necessary at one point in time as a protective defence mechanism. This was based on Pavlov's observation that 'the phenomenon represents a self-protecting reflex of inhibitory character.' From studying dogs, Pavlov recognised that hypnosis is an adaptive response mechanism involving higher nervous activity, evolving to its present form during the course of phylogenetic development.

Hypnosis as a state of hysteria

Hypnosis was once considered as a symptom of hysteria, the theory being that only hysterical individuals were hypnotisable. This theory was discredited because suggestibility was shown not to be an indication of neurosis.

Theories based on changes in cerebral physiology

A number of theories say that hypnosis is due to a changed physiology of the cerebral cortex, an inhibition of the ganglion cells of the brain, the inhibition of one set of mental functions and the excitation of others. Further theories contend that hypnosis is due to a focus of central excitation with surrounding areas of inhibition and, other theories purport that hypnosis is due to synaptic elimination.

Hypnosis as a conditioned process leading to sleep

Evidence has been collated to indicate that hypnosis is due to alterations in the cortical neuron field, principally due to its similarity to sleep. Pavlov said that hypnosis is a partial sleep; he found that the spreading and deepening of localised areas of inhibition through the cortex produced varying degrees of hypnosis. Interestingly, Crailneck and Hall (1985) have been able to convert light sleep into hypnosis; this does not mean, however, that the two are the same. This is also supported by the fact that in normal sleep suggestibility is markedly decreased. This may be due to the fact that rapport is lost, and memories are eradicated.

Kroger (1973) found that a hypnotised person is more aware of his environment than when he is asleep. He states, 'A patient in hypnosis becomes more critical, more articulate. He is not to be thought of as stuporous.'

Ideomotor activity and inhibition theory

Several researchers and authors suggest that the effects of suggestibility are the result of ideomotor action and inhibition. They further suggest that suggestibility is simply the experience of imagining which becomes actualised through ideomotor activities. This, however, fails to account for the complex psychological reactions elicited during hypnosis.

The dissociation theory

According to Kroger (1973), it has been contended for some time that a hypnotised person was in a dissociated state. However, if the dissociated theory were true then amnesia could not be removed by the suggestions of the hypnotist. This theory was abandoned when it was demonstrated that usually instead of amnesia or dissociation during hypnosis, there was hyperacuity and improved co-ordination of all the senses.

The role-playing theory

A widely-held theory in psychology was that someone in hypnosis was playing a role, in other words he behaves as he thinks a hypnotised person should behave. However, the role-playing theory fails to explain how a person's eye pupils can be conditioned to contract involuntarily to a hallucinated light.

The hypersuggestibility theory

This has been a popular theory in the fact that a person's

attention is focused on the hypnotist, and as a result, their suggestions become more effective. This actually fails to explain how hypersuggestibility actually occurs; neither does it explain the spontaneous occurrence of amnesia. This theory also infers that only gullible people are suggestible, whereas my own experience and research suggests that this is not the case.

Miscellaneous theories

One of the theories explored by Klein (1986) suggests that words are represented in our consciousness as symbolic processes to control internal functions, especially those inhibited by the cranial and sacral areas of the autonomic nervous system.

Other theories suggest that hypnosis is due to psychokinetic field forces. Barber (1996) suggests that hypnosis is not a state or a trance, and is not due to subconscious motivation. He states that it is based upon an interpersonal relationship (belief/faith) in which a person's perceptions are restructured, and because the client is inattentive to his environment. This implies that the client is then ready and willing to think as the hypnotist wants him to think. According to Barber, this perceptual-cognitive restructuring is the essential element that creates the hypnosis.

Psychosomatic theories

A complex theory suggests that suggestibility and hypnotic phenomena have a multiple origin based on psychosomatic processes. The basis for this is that suggestibility is an ideomotor action, which is a form of abstract conditioning. This suggests that everything except for the hypnotist's voice is in dissociative awareness; the hypnotist's voice then becomes an extension of the client's own psychic processes. The result is a considerable variety of perceptual changes.

Another theory offered by Crasilneck and Hall (1985), suggests that hypnotic phenomena are due to a psychosomatic reaction comprising a mutual and dynamic interaction of physiological and psychological factors. It states that in a hypnotic relationship the client obtains gratification of earlier dependency needs.

An alternative suggestion (*Kroger, 1973*) is that hypnosis is a specific type function of the ego that is self-excluding. A change occurs from conscious perception to preconscious functioning, similar to the performance of routine activities. This is referred to as topological regression.

The fact that the above remain theories supports the notion that there is a lot more to learn about hypnosis, its uses, and effects. It remains a fascinating course of study, which will no doubt continue for many years while humans attempt to understand the workings of the human mind.

Past Life Regression

The Spirit is the essence of each individual and it cannot be destroyed. The body and its worldly identity are like suits of clothes you exchange as your True Self moves through one manifestation to another.

LaVedi Lafferty & Bud Hollowell,

Eternal Dance; There is no life after death – there is no death 1983

Past life regression is a powerful methodology when used appropriately to enable people to heal dis-ease and trauma from previous lives that manifest in their current life. Interestingly, it has been found by such notable people as Dr. Brian Weiss (2007), that it is not necessary for the client to consciously believe in past lives for the regression process to work. He, and many other therapists specializing in PLR (past life regressions), have successfully regressed numerous people, enabling them to explore past lives in order to understand and heal themselves in this lifetime. In my own practice I often use PLR or Time Line Therapy ™ (see later section) to assist people with healing their lives.

The online encyclopaedia, Wikipedia, a source for a lot of non-academic research (2008), states:

Past Life Regression (PLR) is a therapeutic technique that uses light levels of hypnosis to activate memories, or pseudo-memories that appear to represent past lives. PLR is typically undertaken either in pursuit of a spiritual experience or in a therapeutic setting where it can be used in an attempt to resolve emotional, psychological or psychosomatic problems. Skeptics suggest that the 'memories' are hypnotic confabulations rather than genuine memories of past lives. Some therapists claim that PLR has spiritual and therapeutic value regardless of the empirical validity of the memories.

A personal observation is that this statement brings into light the term psychosomatic, which implies that the dis-ease is all in the mind, therefore created by our thoughts. What I find quite interesting is that this definition implies that some dis-ease is not actually created through the mind – our thoughts. This is counter to much of the emergent thinking which states that dis-ease is created through our thoughts – our mind, and can hence be healed by changing our thoughts. This paper is full of examples of this type of work.

Despite the mixed reviews it receives, PLR has been developed and used by a number of therapists in the USA, UK, and Australia since around 1950. During this time more research has been carried out and published by a number of people. These researchers include Alexander Cannon in 1950 (*The Power Within*), through to Andy Tomlinson in 2006 (*Healing the Eternal Soul*).

In exploring Past Lives, I believe that there are some parallels with the work of Quantum Physicist Niels Bohr. Bohr states that a quantum particle exists as both a wave and a particle, and a wave function. How it exists is related to how the observer expects to see it. Life too exists in this wave form with present, previous, and future lifetimes all on the same wave. The 'I' that exists now is simply a particle on that wave, as are my other lifetimes. We are literally the quantum I and the waves of life!

Reincarnation

The concept of reincarnation is an integral part of the belief systems of a number of religious and spiritual groups around the world. This belief is fundamental to the concept of PLR. Florence Wagner McClain says that the purpose of reincarnation is for us to understand and claim our birthright as an evolving unlimited spirit. This unlimited spirit is created by, and in the image of the ultimate Unlimited Spirit. This realization can be very profound, as it enables us to understand our true nature, to free ourselves from limitations, and accept full responsibility for all our actions. This theosophy goes on to say that once we have achieved this, there is no further need for us to experience any additional lessons attained by a physical existence on this earthly plane.

Reincarnation means different things to different people. However, the simplest definition I have come across (*Wagner McClain, 1986*) is that it is the hypothesis that man's awareness, our soul, survives death, and returns to be born again into a new physical body. This provides us with new opportunities to grow in our knowledge and wisdom. Part of this set of beliefs is that we experience life as both males and females, in numerous races and social standings, encompassing the whole range of good and evil. Therefore, we will experience what it's like to be a slave or a slave owner, a leader and a follower, a wealthy landlord and a serf, a prostitute and a high court judge, and so on. What appear to be important, are not the individual deeds, but the motivation behind them, and whether we choose to grow and learn from these experiences, or not.

Reincarnation is one of the oldest, and fascinatingly, widest-held beliefs around the world. In the beginning of man's life on earth, life was simpler and in tune with the natural cycles of life, death and rebirth. We saw these cycles in nature all around us. It was, therefore, natural for us to believe that we too were part of this eternal cycle, and that our lives would be renewed. Through my research I have found that in the various cultures around the world who continue to live in harmony with nature, there remains a wide-spread belief in reincarnation.

Nevertheless, according to Florence Wagner McClain (1986), we each have both positive and less than positive traits and talents, combined with attitudes that have been developed in previous lifetimes. She says that all of our experiences, both in this life and previous lives, make us who we are today. Furthermore, she says that those who investigate reincarnation through past life regressions are likely to be more acutely aware of the consequences of each thought and action they take, along with the motivations behind these. The realization that our past actions have created the difficult situations and issues we are dealing with now, along with the joy and happiness in ourselves and our lives is a strong incentive to utilize the best within us to create the best of futures for ourselves. This is likely to be much more appealing than the threat of burning in some form of hell and damnation forever.

We may feel that the notion of returning to live again and again is attractive, especially if we have a fear of death. However, as our knowledge and understanding of our cumulative self grows, the prospect of returning time and time again becomes less attractive. Therefore, we will often become more determined to grow and learn as quickly as possible so that we can break the cycle of birth and death.

Transmigration

Transmigration is a term sometimes mixed up with reincarnation. It is the theory that we can come 'back to earth' as a mouse, or a cow, or some other form of life. While I have often heard people talking about this theory, as far as I am aware there appears to be only a few people, mostly in India, who actually believe in this type of incarnation.

Our physical bodies are made up of a variety of communities of living cells, which each perform specific functions, providing a viable host for our souls. To be able to function physically we need a vehicle through which to operate; our physical body. I personally believe that it is highly likely that the theory of transmigration is derived from a metaphor intended to teach humans about our responsibility to all our relations – all life forms. The essence of life that is in every cell of our body comes from the same source, the source that gives life to all living things. Hence, I would also suggest that we should respect our bodies, whether we believe in transmigration or not, as ultimately we are comprised of the stuff of 'all life'.

Memory Recall

PLR is simply a process of tuning in to our unconscious mind to recall memories of past experiences. There are many ways in which we can do this; it can even happen spontaneously, prompted by an event, a place or a person. This actually happened to my husband when we first met. We were sitting together chatting when he spontaneously regressed to a previous lifetime we had shared together. He had been a baker and we had lived in a small village in Medieval Italy. During that lifetime, we had fallen in love, but my parents had arranged for me to marry someone else. He said that he felt that he had lost me and was determined that this wasn't going to happen again this time around.

The regular practice of meditation will often lead to glimpses of past life experiences. Quite often, knowledge and understandings attained in previous lifetimes, are brought into our consciousness. This actually happened to me a week after reading 'Past Life Regressions' by Florence Wagner McClain.

I had been struggling with an issue with my husband and his apparent lack of motivation and stuckness. In my morning meditation I learned that this was all part of his current learning, and this time, my role was simply to be there to love and support him through this phase in his life. It felt like quite a challenge, but one I have become increasingly accepting of as I grow and learn more about myself and life.

Young children often have clear memories of past lives, however, sadly these often fade as they get older, and become more consciously involved in the world. At the age of four, my niece sat on the sofa with my mother and said, 'You know Grandma, Mummy and I were such good friends last time, that this time, I waited until she was ready to have a little girl.' My mother was flabbergasted at the time, however; her beliefs are such that she soon chose to forget about the incident.

Experiences of déjà vu, meaning 'seen before' are sometimes associated with past life memory. Such experiences are those we have when we perceive a sudden feeling that we have been somewhere before, or get a sense that we have had the same conversation on another occasion.

Hypnosis is the most frequently used method for past life regression. It is a very effective method if the hypnotherapist is open to reincarnation. Dr. Brain Weiss was a reluctant convert to hypnosis and past life regression. He was a conventional psychologist, who was working with a client, Catherine, when she spontaneously regressed. This ultimately ignited a spark within him, and he has now used PLR with hundreds of people very successfully, and has written several books on the subject. The most well-known of these is the story of his 'conversion' into believing in PLR with Catherine's story in *Many Lives, Many Masters* (1994). Dr. Weiss states that Catherine changed his life forever by recalling, with stunning accuracy, her travels into past lives, as far apart as the second millennium BCE and the middle of the twentieth century. She reported experiences and descriptions from centuries ago that she could not have known about in this life. These descriptions were validated both by Dr. Weiss, a Yale and Columbia-trained psychologist and other scientists who he engaged in the process.

As Catherine's therapy progressed, she brought back lessons from the Masters (incorporeal guides with great wisdom), who surrounded her when she was in regression. This happened over a quarter of a century ago, and Dr. Weiss now says that these experiences with Catherine, and the wisdom she gleaned, has informed his thoughts and governed his behaviour ever since. She was able to access information through realms that Weiss never knew existed. He was exhilarated, astonished and scared simultaneously. He was also concerned that if he shared his experiences he would be cast out of the psychological community. During the intervening years, Dr. Weiss has regressed more than four thousand people. In *Many Lives, Many Masters* (1994), he says that his confidence grew with the increasing numbers of people he was able to help with PLR. He was also encouraged by the fact that other professionals were also experiencing similar results using PLR techniques.

In the last few years Dr Weiss has been developing an approach to progression therapy. On occasion during the last twenty-five years he has had patients who have spontaneously progressed into a future life. This has usually happened towards the end of their therapy. If he felt confident of their ability to understand that what they were witnessing may be fantasy, he would encourage them to go on, saying something like, 'This is about growth and experiencing, helping you now to make proper and wise decisions. But we are going to avoid any memories, (memories of the future), visions, or connections with any death scenes or serious illnesses. This is only for learning' (*Weiss*, 2007). He found that these people were able to make wiser decisions and better choices. They could look at a near-future event and make choices about which path to take, and sometimes their look at the future would come true.

Karma

Through his work in regression and progression, Dr. Weiss came to learn that past, present, and future are one, and that what happens in the future can influence the present, just as the past influences it. This concept is supported by the work of Daniel Everett, (2008) who has lived with a tribe in the Amazon for more than 25 years. The tribe, the Piraha, believe that there is only now, that past, present and future all happen simultaneously. Dr Weiss further theorizes that as we have an apparent limitless number of past lives, the same could be said about future lives. So, by using our knowledge of what went before and what is to come, we might be able to shape the world's future and our futures. This reflects the ancient concept of karma.

There is much written about karma, which is in essence the law of cause and effect. Florence Wagner McClain (1986), states that the purpose of karma is to teach us, and to help us learn to live in harmony with the universe. It is not a punitive process as thought by many people. Cause and effect is a Universal Law, meaning that for every action (cause), there is a reaction (effect). Much of what goes on around us we cannot control; however, we can choose which actions or causes we set into motion, and the attitude we take to deal with the effects of these actions. It is our attitudes that create the karma into favourable or unfavourable influences in our lives. Karma simply is. It is of itself neither positive, nor negative.

I often hear people talking about karmic debt as in suffering, or the reason for some unpleasant aspect of their lives. It is rare that people focus on, or talk about the knowledge, wisdom, skills, talents, friends, and loved ones which are the outcomes of past life experiences, and therefore also a part of our karmic heritage. To illustrate, we can use a simple example of shoes; if we wear shoes that are too small, our feet will hurt. This is cause and effect, the effect is that our feet hurt, and the cause is that the shoes are too small. We have a choice as to how we deal with the situation. We can continue to wear the shoes, be in pain, and no doubt be miserable and grumpy, and there is even the possibly that we cause some permanent damage to our feet. Alternatively, we can learn from the experience, give the shoes away, and wear some more comfortable shoes. This then allows us to focus on the important things in life. In a nutshell, this is karma.

The most popular belief about karma is that we must suffer in this life if we have caused someone else to suffer in a past life. I am unsure as to the purpose of such thoughts. What would be the purpose? How does creating more suffering in this world help us or anyone else?

One of our fundamental learnings in our spiritual evolvement is that karma is essentially a learning experience for gaining wisdom. It is not a system of punishment and reward. We use our free will to choose the learnings that will be of most benefit to others and ourselves. Our instinct, skills, and talents, which successfully guide us through new or challenging circumstances, and self-confidence, are all results of our past actions. Over our eons of living we have gained a vast repertoire of expertise and knowledge in many, many areas of life. All this knowledge of multiple successes and failures is available to us, and so can be retrieved for use in our present life simply through regression.

We are continually dealing with the law of cause and effect when dealing with the effects of other people's actions. The choice here is about how we decide to let their actions affect us. Essentially, karma is about accepting personal responsibility for our lives, and fundamental to that is our attitude. We actually do what we really want to do. This can be a 'hard pill to swallow' as it means that we accept personal responsibility for the current condition of our lives. In accepting this we can no longer blame situations, other people or karma for the circumstances of our lives, and we are free to change things through the act of free will.

The Process of Regression

When working with clients, it is fundamentally important to choose a place where the 'client' feels comfortable both physically and mentally, and where you will not be interrupted. I have a room I call the 'Imaginarium' that I work in, which is dedicated to therapy and healing. I ask my client to take off their shoes, and recline or sit in a comfortable position. I have a light blanket nearby, which is useful to have at hand as people's temperatures can shift during a session. Having a bathroom close by is also important, as I have found that hypnosis works at particular levels of mental activity which seem to speed up bodily functions.

People being regressed are often vulnerable to the mental and emotional attitudes of those around them. Therefore, it is really important to keep the energy of the room light and up beat, and to clear my mind before I start working with people. A sense of humour can also help to ease any tension, and avoid any feelings that make the process feel like a test. I have found that it is important to emphasise that we are simply recalling memories from the distant past, and there is no right or wrong, success or failure to this process. Different people will naturally recall different levels of detail, just as we do when we are recalling early childhood memories. This is perfectly natural, and it is important to stress that the information gleaned should be accepted without judgement.

I find that taking notes is a helpful way to jog memories afterwards, and to identify patterns over a number of regressions, which may be helpful to healing a present life situation.

Sensory Acuity

In the work I have done myself along with the people I have

trained in hypnotherapy, I know that it is important for the regressor/hypnotherapist to remain aware and observant throughout the session. It is vitally important to watch for specific signs of significant stress or tension. This is usually seen as:

Agitated hand movements,

Clenched jaw,

Clenched fists,

Uncontrollable laughter,

Tears combined with any of the other signs. Tears alone are usually a sign of a healthy catharsis, and can often be appropriate to the particular incident.

If the therapist is faced with any of the above situations, the best action to take is to calmly ask if something is bothering their client and would they like to end the regression now or go on to something else. It is often helpful to remind them that they are 'here and now', that this is only a recalled memory, and that there is no need to feel any kind of pain or distress.

If the person being regressed says that they wish to end the session, the therapist will gently bring the person out of the regressed state and repeat the positive statements above. If on the other hand they want to continue, the therapist will give instructions to progress to a different time (a week, month, year ahead, whichever feels appropriate), and proceed. Once the session is complete, I suggest that the therapist discusses the incident that caused the emotional response. This is helpful in enabling the 'regressee' (regressed person) to identify how this memory may play out in their current life.

Releasing Judgement

It is fundamentally important for the regressee to be able to relax and remember that this is simply an exercise in memory recall; hence there are no right or wrong answers. They should answer any questions with the first thoughts that come to mind no matter how they may feel about the thought. It is also important that they do not attempt to analyse their answers or align them with accepted thinking or historically known facts. The reason behind this is that in many instances information that may seem to be at variance with recorded history often proves to be accurate. Interestingly, in many instances, recorded history is markedly different from what actually happened at the time, this is due to the fact that it has been influenced by the feelings and prejudices of the writer.

I always instruct the regressee to accept the information in whichever way it comes as it can be received in a number of ways. Some people feel as if they are re-living the experience, and participating in it fully, others feel as if they are simply an observer watching the story unfold. Yet others have very few if any, visual impressions, instead they will hear, smell, feel, or get a general sense of what is going on. I always emphasise that whichever way the information is retrieved is perfect.

I also find that it is important to inform the regressee that regression is really a way of getting to know oneself. It is an opportunity to learn to become sensitive to subtle changes in their senses and body during regression sessions. If for example, the regressee is in a large city and becomes aware of a farmyard smell during the regression, it may be useful to assume that they are in or near a farmyard in their past life time. This level of sensitivity helps to focus their mind on that particular lifetime which usually becomes easier with each subsequent regression.

The person being regressed should also know that there is very little about the regression experience that is really crucial. For example, it is ok for them to change their posture allowing themselves to be more comfortable. They should also know that they are in control, and can end the session whenever they want to. I tell them that the only important thing to remember in prematurely ending a session is to ensure that they affirm to themselves something like, 'I will bring with me all information and impressions that are of benefit to me, and I leave behind anything which is of detriment to me.'

Finally, it is important that no mind-altering drugs or alcohol are taken prior to a session as they are likely to distort the experience.

Relaxation

Set out below is an example of the kind of relaxation process I will commonly use when undertaking a regression session:

'Ok, now I want you to relax, take a few long deep breaths and begin to feel yourself relaxing. Now, close your eyes and feel your eyelids relaxing, with each breath feel those eyelids relaxing more and more (pause). Breathe the relaxation into any of the little muscles around your eyes that feel any tension, just let that tension go now (pause), make them relax.

'Now focus your attention on your scalp (pause), breathe the relaxation into all the tiny muscles on your scalp, feel them relaxing (pause). Feel each of those muscles as they relax completely, now. Feel the relaxation across your scalp.

'Now move your attention to your face (pause), breathe relaxation into all of the muscles of your face. Relax all of those muscles (pause), feel them relax completely.

'Next, focus your attention on your jaw (pause), our jaws hold lots of tension, so, breathe the relaxation into those muscles, feel them relax (pause), scan these muscles for tension, and cause them to relax.

'Now (pause), focus on your neck (pause), breathe the relaxation into your neck muscles and along your shoulders, feel them relax now (pause). Feel each muscle relax, let them relax; allow your neck and shoulders to relax completely.

'Next bring your attention to your hands (pause), feel the relaxation move down your arms and into your hands. Become aware of all of the small muscles in your hands and fingers, and feel them relax more with each breath (pause). Allow your hands and fingers to relax completely.

'Now focus your attention on your chest (pause), this area contains muscles, organs, nerves and glands. Breathe the relaxation into this area (pause), feel your chest relaxing, every muscle, every organ, every nerve and every gland, just feel the tension ebb away as they relax (pause). Allow every cell in your chest to function in a natural, rhythmic manner (pause), allow your chest to completely relax.

'Now move your attention to your abdomen (pause), this area contains muscles, organs, nerves and glands. Breathe the relaxation into this area (pause), feel your abdomen relaxing, every muscle, every organ, every nerve and every gland, just feel the tension ebb away as they relax (pause). Allow every cell in your chest to function in a natural, rhythmic manner (pause). Allow your abdomen to completely relax.

'Next shift your attention to your legs (pause), breathe relaxation into each of the muscles in your legs, simply allow them to relax (pause). Feel your legs relax (pause), allow them to relax completely.

'Next bring your attention to your feet (pause), feel the relaxation move down your legs and into your feet. Become aware of all of the small muscles in your feet and toes and feel them relax more with each breath (pause). Allow your feet and toes to relax completely.

'Relaxation is natural; it is a wonderful feeling, a healthy way of being. Anytime you want to return to this state (pause) of relaxation, simply take a deep breath, and as you exhale say the word 'relax' to yourself three times, and you will once again be completely relaxed.'

Safety

If a client asks to be regressed for a specific problem it is important to instruct them to, 'Go to the point in time that is the root cause of this problem.' It is important that prior to such a specific regression the client has already had some experience with regressions and is comfortable with the process. This should only be done with the explicit understanding that if the problem is distressing in this lifetime it has the potential for being amplified at the time of its root cause. It is therefore also important to reassure the client periodically throughout the regression that they are simply going through a process of remembering. Remind them that they are physically here and now, and emphasise that there is no need for them to experience any distress at any level. It is also helpful to encourage them to dissociate as if they were watching the scene on a television or at the movies. If my client finds it difficult to dissociate I will combine this with Time Line Therapy ™ (see later) to facilitate their dissociation from the feelings and release the root cause.

Phobias

It is generally accepted by the psychological community that the more common problems that we face in our lives are associated with a form of fear, and sometimes these fears can escalate into phobias. One definition of a phobia is, 'a seemingly irrational and persistent fear which is socially paralysing. Reactions which are abnormal and out of proportion to the threat (if any) presented are consistently triggered by the same object, event, environment or person' (*Wagner McClain, 1986 p. 87*).

One example is when I was having a conversation with a young client in my 'Imaginarium'. I noticed that he suddenly recoiled in horror when I used a cigarette lighter to light a candle. He told me that he lived in fear of fire, and that if anyone lit a candle or struck a match in his presence he would panic, tremble and perspire, often running from the room in fright. Neither he nor his parents could recall any childhood trauma which would account for this seemingly irrational fear.

I conducted a regression with this young man and discovered

that in his most recent past life he had burned to death in a house fire. Thankfully, using the positive statements in the closing of the regression technique removed most of the trauma. We later discussed the process, and I reassured him that the circumstances from his previous life were unlikely to recur. He said that he felt a huge burden had been lifted from his mind during the regression; then he asked me for a lighter. He took a deep breath and ignited the lighter, as he did so a broad smile lit up his face. He later attended one of my fire walking training events and laughed happily as he walked over the hot coals.

A second example is of a friend who had a spider phobia. She was sitting in my living room having a cup of tea, while we chatted about her future plans for a holiday with her young son. Suddenly she started to choke; shake and turned ashen. After a while she calmed down, and told me that she had seen a spider rush across the living room floor. She had this phobia for as long as she could remember, and she asked me if I would do a regression for her. I regressed her to a time when she had been a nomad traversing the Sahara when she had been bitten by a large tarantula type of spider. As a result, in that lifetime she had died a painful and traumatic death, alone in the desert.

A month or so later she was once again at my home when she saw another spider. I had actually seen it before her and was curious to see her response. She simply laughed and said, 'Do you actually create these spiders for me when I come to your house?'

These examples indicate to me the usefulness of regression techniques for many life situations.

Choice

We can also glean insights into the purpose of choosing our parents, and the lessons we can learn from them, along with the full blueprint we have created for this lifetime through regression. (The blueprint enables us to fix into our awareness that which we wished to accomplish in this lifetime.) We may even find that we have already achieved much of what we intended, if this is the case we are free to identify a new set of goals. Maybe this information will help us to find answers to some of our current frustrations.

Alternatively, we may discover that we have deviated from our blueprint, and the things we wanted to achieve. This is often manifested as little naggings and feelings that we are not really satisfied with our direction. If this is the case, it is useful to ask ourselves some questions like, 'Has the deviation taken me in a positive and fruitful direction?' Alternatively, 'Is the deviation my own choice or was it as a result of someone else's actions over which I had no apparent control?'

It is also possible that others made choices that changed the circumstances of our environment, either between the time we chose our parents and were born, or possibly even at later times. If we find that the direction of our lives is beneficial despite the deviation, it is helpful to mentally affirm that we are letting go of the original blueprint. This enables us to follow a direction that is more appropriate to us now, and hence release a number of our naggings and frustrations.

One theory (*Wagner McClain , 1986*) is that if we find that we have deviated from our original blueprint without any real reason, we should look at that blueprint to identify the changes we need to make to progress our spiritual growth. We may find that there are compromises we need to make to alter our course, depending upon how far along we are in this lifetime. A balanced assessment may show us that it is not necessarily the choices we have made, but how we make them that is important. The attitudes we choose in our lives will often make the difference as to how out of kilter or harmony we are with our blueprint. To succeed with this, we need to rehearse success in our minds, and to cultivate a sense of fairness, tolerance and kindness to ourselves and others. By holding an image of ourselves acting and reacting with the qualities we aspire to, we will soon find that these become a part of our lives. As someone once said to me, our blueprint is: 'More a set of guidelines than tram lines.'

Learning

Our minds are programmed to seek solutions to problems, so whether we choose to believe in past lives or merely see regression as an exercise of a vivid imagination, the mind uses this to solve our problems. Regression promotes a social understanding and tolerance of the opposite sex, other cultures or races, and aids us in becoming more balanced and whole. It actually opens a door to accepting and understanding our personal responsibility, and helps us to rid ourselves of unnecessary and unhealthy feelings. Our personal relationships often benefit as we develop a deeper insight into our own nature.

Regression enables us to identify the role or situation to remember which best suits our current situation or stage of learning. This occurs at the deep Alpha levels of our consciousness, in our unconscious mind. It enables us to release fear, guilt and other negative feelings, the effect of which is immediate and real. Regression also provides a healthy way to release our anger, stresses, and frustrations, hence improving our well-being both now and in the future. This in itself enables us to be more relaxed about life, and the challenges with which it presents us. Combine this with the fact that regression opens a door to infinite possibilities for finding very practical and useful information, and we find we have an invaluable tool to improve our lives easily and with little effort.

Again, according to Florence Wagner McClain (1986), 'We are each personally responsible for the role which we play in the destiny of our civilisation.' This is a very profound statement as few people would allow themselves to consider this possibility. She is proposing that we should be willing to take the time and make the effort to understand our previous lifetimes in relation to our present selves. This can also provide us with information about how our behaviours and attitudes have each contributed to the rise and fall of each civilisation we have lived in.

The message I receive from this is that regression is a useful tool to better understand ourselves, and gives us the ability to take a long hard look at the social consciousness that we have demonstrated in our previous lives. It also gives us the opportunity to ask ourselves some potentially hard questions. Did we go along with the crowd because it was easy, or did we stand up against the injustices with wisdom; did we take immature action escalating the problems? Did we allow care and concern for others to motivate us or not? Were there times when we behaved arrogantly towards others, and lifetimes when we were kindly and supportive? Did we make decisions that brought destruction or help to strengthen and grow a balanced society? Were there times when we were timid or brave, wealthy or poor, lazy or active?

The law of cause and effect has a direct impact on the progress and benefits we enjoy today. In other words the decisions we made in our 'yesterdays' affect our 'todays' both for us individually and as a society. Once I realised this, it began to have a significant impact on the daily choices I make, such as, from decisions about how much water I use to do the laundry or clean my teeth, to how I choose to do 'my work' in the world. This is because we truly do have a personal responsibility for the roles that *we choose* to play in the destiny of our civilisations.

Time Transformation Techniques (T3)

The Origins

Time Transformation Techniques (T3), have their roots in NLP (Neuro Linguistic Programming). A substantial number of the deeper processes in NLP induce ASCs to facilitate change, and many of these ASCs are attained through a trans-derivational search (TDS). This is when a client has to search through the various different modalities to find an answer to a question, and is seen when their eyes move through all four accessing quadrants. This happens when the question presented is plausible to the unconscious mind, and yet there is no automatic answer. So, the client has to search for the information which results in a brief ASC, and provides the opportunity to access the unconscious mind where change can take place.

NLP was first conceived in the 1970s By Richard Bandler and John Grinder. They were intrigued by the impact of communication, and how some people were able to excel in communication and others not. They studied the ways in which great communicators, such as Milton Erickson and Virginia Satir amongst others, were able to work with people to facilitate desired change. From their immaculate work and attention to detail, NLP as we know it today was born.

Time Line Therapy™ is a process that was originally conceived by Tad James and Wyatt Woodsmall. They published their work in 1988 in a book entitled, *Time Line Therapy and the Basis of Personality.* This methodology provides us with a combination of processes that enable us to understand and use core aspects of a person's personality in creating healing.

The essential NLP components expanded in TLT (Time Line Therapy™) are Time Line (memory storage), Metaprograms, and Values. This built on the original knowledge of how people store memories along with the way in which the mechanisms used to store these memories have an impact on the personality of the individual.

The authors contend that the notion of time we have stored in our minds both shape and structure our experience of the world. Metaprograms are the most basic filters that process the sensory data that we receive from the outside world. The third component, Values, also serve as a filtering mechanism in the processing of sensory data. They are in fact the most basic of the filters that have content in and of themselves. Our Values are even more basic than our beliefs, and supply the energy behind our motivation, providing the selection criteria for our strategies. Our Values are how we assess right and wrong, and are the basis for how we evaluate our behaviour.

The concept of the linear storage of time has a long history, dating back to Aristotle who talked about 'the stream of time'. The ancient Greeks also had two separate concepts of time, one describing the qualitative aspects (Karios) as an internal expression, and one describing the quantitative aspects (Chronos) as an external expression. Closer to our present day, in 1982 Leslie Cameron Bandler ran a workshop where she discussed the concepts of 'in-time' (associated) and 'through time' (dissociated) memory storage. This stimulated the modern day use of time lines and TLT. After being influenced by Leslie Cameron Bandler, Steve and Connirae Andreas, Anne Linden and Frank Stass, Wyatt Woodsmall began teaching about time lines in his NLP Practitioner and Master Practitioner trainings in 1985.

In 1985 Tad and Ardie James attended the NLP trainings given by Wyatt Woodsmall. Wyatt discussed his work on time lines, and this intrigued Tad and Marvin Oka who began to experiment with both the therapeutic and the personal growth applications. This work lead to collaboration between Wyatt and Tad which resulted in the publication of *Time-Line Therapy and the Basis of Personality* (1988).

Process Development

In 2002, after studying TLT with Tad James, and Meta-States ® with L. Michael Hall, my husband Robert Moeller and I developed a process that combines both methodologies into one process. This is known as Time Transformation Techniques (T3). We had both found TLT to be the most effective method for enabling clients to release their anchors to past experiences and to move forward in their lives. However, it soon became apparent that whilst it was very beneficial to enable people to remove these memories from their lives, it often left a void. It is a well-known concept that life abhors a vacuum, and so we became aware that in all likelihood these gaps would be filled in a relatively arbitrary manner. We therefore sought to find a way to fill this gap more consciously with something that was supportive and positive; hence we found an effective way to combine the TLT process with an element of Meta-States ® (MS).

To use a gardening analogy, our minds are just like gardens. If we pull out all the weeds, and then don't plant the seeds of the plants we desire, the likelihood is that we will get more weeds. The seed for those weeds can fall from the sky thanks to birds flying overhead, or drop off animals walking through our garden, or even be carried in by the winds of time. If you are a gardener, you will know that if you plant your seeds, tend, and nurture them, keeping any new weeds at bay, in a very short time the seeds that you planted will grow. Given time those seeds will grow big enough and strong enough to keep most new weeds at bay. As a result of planting and nurturing those seeds, they will develop deep strong roots, building up resistance to many different kinds of pest. Those same seeds will also begin a process by which they will self-generate, where you will have all you want, and you will be able to share your good fortune with others.

In the T3 methodologies, once the negative emotions are released, we plant the seeds of desired 'positive' emotions and resourceful states, along with the openness and flexibility to realise the benefit in all our emotions. I feel it is important to note at this time that when we make the distinction between positive and negative emotions, we know that this is subjective and arguably there is no such thing as positive or negative emotions. However, for the purposes of training people at this particular level we identify positive emotions as those that bring peace, calmness, and flexibility into our lives, and those that do not, as negative emotions. We also teach that our negative emotions, when understood and befriended can assist us in realising where we have gone adrift.

The Storage of Time

The first step in this process is to elicit a person's timeline. People usually store time as in the diagram below,

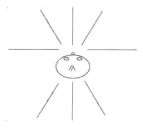

Figure 4: Eliciting someone's timeline (from AND Master Practitioner Manual 1996)

The people whose timelines go through their bodies are designated 'in-time'. These people are fully associated with the moment of now, they may find it challenging to plan ahead, and can easily lose themselves in a task without any awareness of time. People whose timelines are in front or beside them are known as 'meta-time', this is a redesignation of the original concept of 'through time', these people are dissociated from their timeline and view it from a meta perspective. They find it easy to plan ahead and see a process from beginning to end; they also remember when things happened in the past with ease.

The simplest way to elicit someone's timeline is to ask, 'If I were to ask your unconscious mind where your past is, and where your future is, I suspect that your unconscious... mind would indicate some linear orientation indicating a line with some orientation relative to your body. So, if I were to ask your unconscious... mind what direction would your past be, what direction would you point?'

'And your future, what direction would you point to indicate that, if I were to ask your unconscious?' (*Andreas, C & S, 1988*).

It is also important to use sensory acuity as often people will say they don't know where their timeline is, and yet their eyes or head will move in a particular direction giving us a clue as to the direction of their timeline. It is then simply a matter of identifying whether the line goes through the person or beside them in some way.

Identifying a Root Cause

Once the client's timeline is elicited, it is important to identify the root cause of their particular problem. This is achieved as follows:

Step 1 Pre-framing is important, so we ask, 'Is it alright with your unconscious mind for you to release this (emotion/limiting decision) today, and for you to be aware of it consciously?'

Step 2 Discovery phase, where we ask the client to identify the mental-emotional state(s) that they want to develop muscle memory of. We then amplify and anchor the emotions (breaking state between each state and at the end of this step). This enables the client to understand at a physical level the mental-emotional state they wish to feel instead of the current re-action to the circumstances we wish to change.

Step 3 Identifying the first event, we ask 'What is the root cause of this problem, the first event which, when disconnected, will cause the problem to disappear?'

'If you were to know, was it before, during, or after your birth?'

If they reply before, we ask, 'In the womb or before?'

If they reply in the womb, we ask, 'What month?'

If they reply before, we ask, 'Was it past life or passed down genealogically?'

If they reply, past life, we ask, 'How many lifetimes ago?'

If they reply genealogical, we ask, 'How many generations ago?'

If they reply after, we ask, 'If you were to know, what age were you?' (8)

These questions are designed to create a brief ASC as the client has usually not experienced such questions before, and has to do a TDS to access the information, resulting in a light trance.

This is also often the first time someone has been asked if their issue is the result of something in a previous life. I find that most times, although not exclusively, people will identify an age in this lifetime when they first experienced TLT or T3. With repetition, when they feel more comfortable with the process, they often move into healing 'stuff' from previous lives. This is the way it happened for me, after a number of TLT 'regressions' I was able to move further back into previous lives, and heal both genealogical and past life manifestations in this life.

An overview of the complete methodology

The T3 methodology is an excellent form of brief therapy, combining TLT with some of the Meta States work of L. Michael Hall. Hence the following script is an adaptation of the original TLT script taught to me by Tad James in 1996. Through the elimination of negative emotions and limiting decisions the space is created for the installation of the desired positive resourceful states, enabling our clients to client-create an empowering future.

Take a detailed Personal History. This is important in eliciting as much information as possible to ensure that we have all the information needed to facilitate our client in releasing the emotion or decision that is holding them back.

Pre-Frame the intervention. This enables us to describe to the client the role of their unconscious mind in keeping the body healthy and whole. We also explain that negative emotions or limiting decision may have had a purpose in the original event, but that they have now become redundant.

Elicit the client's timeline orientation and note the direction.

Facilitate the client in floating up above their timeline. The purpose of this is to familiarise the client with their timeline, and to have them undertake a test run into the past, future, and way up very high. In doing this the client is entering into an ASC, and remains in some level of ASC until we reach the final step.

Elicit the sub-modalities of the timeline. While the client is floating way up very high, elicit the visual sub-modalities of the timeline. This enables us to gauge any changes once the work is complete.

Elicit the root cause of the negative emotions/limiting decisions. This step is fundamentally important to the success of the whole process.

Check that it is ok with the client's unconscious mind to release the negative emotions/limiting decisions and to be aware of it consciously. This helps to eliminate any secondary gain.

Preserve the learnings. During T3 processes we guide and facilitate the client in learning from the experience. It is important to remember that learnings are positive, about the person themselves and future orientated.

Release the negative emotions/limiting decisions. After identifying the root cause and checking the ecology of the proposed change work, we guide the client above their timeline and into the past, where we do the actual healing work. The basic steps are: a) locating the event, b) preserving the learnings, c) releasing the emotion, and d) testing that the emotion/decision has been released.

Install the positive resourceful states. Here we guide our client to install the positive emotion(s) and resourceful state(s) that they had previously identified with which they would like to replace the old emotion.

Make the necessary emotional changes to the person's life history. After the client has released the negative emotions, they are guided to stop at every event between then and now to release the emotion and preserve the learnings. The purpose for this is to clean up any remnants of the unwanted emotion.

Return the client to the present moment. Break State.

Future Pace. This is where we guide our client into the future, and have them imagine a similar event that previously would have caused the problem state to appear. We have them notice how differently they respond now.

Check Ecology. Here we once again check for an honest unconscious indication of whether or not there is any thing else to do.

Bring the client's awareness back into the room.

Most people say something like, 'Wow that was amazing, it has really gone!'

Of all of the sets of tools in my repertoire this is the set I use most frequently. This is a simple and yet highly effective use of ASC to guide a client into health and healing, and one that is a daily part of my healing and therapy practice.

Chapter V

Shamanistic Practices of Using ASCs

The Australian Aborigines and indeed indigenous tribal peoples all over the world believe that the spirit of their consciousness and way of life exists like a seed buried in the earth. The waves of European colonialism that destroyed the civilisations of North America, South America, and Australia began a five hundred-year dormancy period of the 'archaic consciousness.' Its potencies disappeared into the earth.

Dreams, deep collective memories and imaginings are more potent than religious faith or scientific theories in lifting us above the catastrophic ending that confronts us all.

Robert Lawlor, Voices of the First Day:
Awakening the Aboriginal Dreamtime 1991.

Five years ago, my husband and I were invited to host two South American Shamans who were spending time in Europe running healing sessions. In the early hours one summer morning, we drove across country to Luton airport to collect them. When we arrived we had no difficulty identifying our guests, as two out of the four were dressed in traditional Peruvian attire. One brief look and I instinctively knew that something in my life was going to change as a result of their visit.

Don Ramon was a delightfully mischievous, 84 year-old from the high Andes, he spoke Quechua and a little broken Spanish. When I asked him how he came to be involved in this work in Europe, he told me a story that rocked me to the core. One of my teachers, Peggy, had been taking groups of people to visit Don Ramon in the high Andes for several years. During one of her visits, he told her that he had been given a message by Pachamama (Mother Earth). He was told that it was now time to reveal the old ways and to teach the people of the west, those who would listen and teach others about Pachamama, and how to live in balance with her, rather than destroy her. The people of the world needed to know how to heal her to save mankind as a whole. He had known for some time that he would be called upon to something outside of his own community, and that would take all his courage, but at the age of 84 he was still surprised at the request. He had never left his homeland of the mountains; however, he knew it was important that he honour this request. He knew he had to offer the people who are destroying the world through their materialism an opportunity to learn a different way, a way of honour and balance.

So after a three-day walk down the mountains to catch a bus, followed by a two-day drive into Lima and a long transatlantic flight, ending in a four-hour drive to our home, this gentle and powerful shaman found himself sitting on my living room floor. He was conducting a ceremony to link the spirits of the land of my home to those of the land of his own.

I was enthralled by both his courage and his story. This lovely octogenarian was prepared to venture into this strange land to help people he had never met, to heal both their lives and that of the planet. In our western culture, most people of his age are seen as being in the twilight of their lives, a time to do very little. I wonder how many of them would truly contemplate such a personal sacrifice as Don Ramon was making on our behalf. The remainder of the shamans' visit was illuminating in many ways. I learned many things about healing and balance, but the biggest gift for me was the realization that someone was prepared to sacrifice so much so that we in the west could be given the opportunity to learn how to use our states of consciousness to heal ourselves, and our planet. I was deeply touched, and so I began a new phase of my own learning and development into Shamanism.

In his book, *The World Is As You Dream It* (1996), John Perkins describes a similar personal experience. He describes how he was visiting Numi, a Shuar shaman. They were talking about the destruction of the rainforests and their people when John asked Numi what he, John, could do to help. The answer he received surprised him, 'If you want to help us,' he said slowly and deliberately, 'if you want to help these forests, then you should start with your own people. It is your people more than mine that need to change.' John understood, and then asked him how he could help, the answer he received shocked him. 'Bring people. Bring your people to us. We can help change that dream you have of huge factories, tall buildings and more automobiles than there are grains of sand.' Shortly thereafter, John began taking groups of people who wanted to learn how to change the dream of the west, to learn from the Shuar and other indigenous groups in Ecuador.

I have also spoken to Native American people who say that now is the time for the old ways to re-emerge. What I understand from this is that we need to come out of the dream, (the 'asleep' state of consciousness) which focuses on materialism and move into a more balanced consciousness of living in tune with our surroundings. We need to develop a relationship of 'give and take', rather than 'take and take', a relationship that invests in the future, our future and the future of our children and their children.

What Is Shamanism?

Shamanism is very probably the oldest known spiritual discipline in the world; it has been an integral part of all hunter/gatherer cultures around the world for millennia. Signs of shamanic practice have been discovered in places as diverse as Australia, the Americas, Siberia, and Europe dating back to prehistory. The world is full of rock paintings, carvings, and painted shells, which give us glimpses into the lives of the shaman over many centuries. When I visited the Tassili Plateau in Algeria we were shown rock paintings of what appeared to be men in space helmets as well as pictorial stories of hunts and star travel.

Shamanism is about a range of spiritual practices which cut across all faiths and creeds, reaching deep levels of ancestral and universal memory. It is neither a religion nor a cult as it is inherently found across the globe. It is a belief system that precedes established religion, with its own universal symbolism and cosmology, inhabited by beings, gods and totems who all display similar characteristics, although they appear in various forms, depending on the beliefs of the people and their geography.

The word shaman, (saman) is taken from the Tungus tribe of the Altai Mountains of Siberia (*Matthews,* 1991). Variations of this word are used in the many cultures around the world to describe someone who through trance and a state of ecstasy, enters into other states of being to that in which he or she usually lives, returning with news from which we can all (humanity) benefit. Shaman can be translated as meaning 'to burn up, to set on fire', referring to the shaman's ability to work with the energy of heat. This is the same skill which enables firewalkers to remain unhurt and yogis to sit naked in the snow for several days without dying of hypothermia; this is possible through their understanding and manipulation of the energies and temperatures of the body. In the twilight place of non-being, between the worlds, the insights, wisdom, and understanding of the shaman are born.

Other meanings of the word shaman are 'one who is excited, moved, raised up.' This can also be traced to the Indo-European root word meaning 'to know', or sometimes 'to heat oneself'. At its foundation the word refers to what its most famous explorer, Mircea Eliade (1972) refers to as 'an archaic technique of ecstasy'; a way of perceiving our place in creation, and of finding the active role we play within it. The emphasis here is on the word *active;* Shamans continually work on themselves to develop improved and more lasting ways to interact with, and encounter the dimensions of the sacred.

Therefore, the shaman acts as a conduit between his or her people and the 'other worlds'. Whilst there are no direct comparisons within our present culture, he or she is seen as a medicine person, priest, and, or healer. Going into an ASC, often described as ecstatic trance, is an integral part of shamanic practice. Shamans will go into trance through a variety of methods such as forms of self-hypnosis, repetitive drumming and the use of hallucinogenic plants. The use of hallucinogenic plant medicine is central to most shamanic traditions. In the Amazon, the most notable of these is Ayahuasca, a complex brew with renowned healing properties. In North America, tobacco and peyote are used, and in Siberia, marijuana is smoked. The use of these substances is so central to Shamanic practices that some researchers, such as the late Terrence McKenna (1992), believe that they are inextricably linked with the origins of human spirituality. Additionally, there are traces of hallucinogenic plant use in almost all historical religions, a curious fact that is largely ignored by most modern religions.

A shaman is essentially a master of energy and its use. By the use of a range of practices, he or she is able to diagnose and cure disease. Shamans have also been credited with the ability to control the weather, divination, the interpretation of dreams, astral projection, and travel to upper and lower worlds. Shamanism is based on the premise that invisible forces or spirits that affect the lives of the living pervade the visible world.

A quick search on the internet demonstrates how popular shamanism has become, with schools for shamanic studies and trips into remote parts of the world to meet shamans fast becoming the latest fad for the 'in crowd'. My concern with this is that it potentially fosters an environment for imposters and people who want to make a quick buck.

A process called journeying is known to be common to all

shamanic cultures. The 'journey' is undertaken by a shaman on behalf of his client to retrieve a lost part of the person's soul or to get some advice on the type of plants to use that will enable healing to take place. The shaman goes into an ASC, facilitated by a monotonous drumbeat. This sound enables the shaman to connect with the spirit of the universe and to retrieve any knowledge vital for healing. This is what is known as shamanic journeying. (See later.)

In India, the Sora believes that the shaman commands his soul to leave his body in order to meet with the spirits, and they can speak through him. In Siberia, the shaman takes flight to the other world where he meets spirit teachers and can rescue lost souls. In Haiti, the soul of the shaman goes to primal Africa, so that ancestors and angel-like beings can take over his body and transmit their healing through him. Journeying is therefore seen as a means for exploring the spiritual universe, making contact with tutelary spirits, recovering lost energy and finding out more about ourselves and our purpose.

Women are often powerful shamans; however menstruating women do not participate in ceremonies. This is due to the fact that menstruation creates changes in hormonal balance, and the subtle effects of these shifts can alter the trance of people around them. Hence, women shamans really come into their full power after they have gone through what we in the west call the menopause. These women, often known as crones are truly powerful shamans with great wisdom.

In his ground breaking work in the 1950s, Mircea Eliade found that many cultures shared similar characteristics. He argued that many of the themes of Siberian shamanism also appeared in other cultures, from India and Tibet through Japan across the Bering Strait to North and South America. He devoted his life to this work and has become the grandfather of this field of study.

The whole concept of Shamanism is to leave the strict world of ego-consciousness and enter the world of the Unconscious, and by doing so gain access to higher consciousness (which ego-consciousness has no direct access to). In this respect it has the same foundation as Hypnosis.

Shamanic Journeying

When people begin to journey to non ordinary reality, they often wonder, 'Am I making this up?' Society as it is today would respond, yes. A shaman would say, 'Did you see it, or hear it, or feel it, or smell it?' If one answers yes, a shaman's reply would be, 'Well, what's wrong with you that you think you're making it up?'
Sandra Ingerman, Soul Retrieval, 1991

At the heart of many shamanic practices is a process called shamanic journeying. This is where the shaman will 'journey' to other realities by attaining altered states of consciousness, and travel outside of time to hidden realms that seem non-ordinary. These realities are deemed parallel to our own. The Australian Aborigines call this reality 'dreamtime', and the Celtic traditions call it the 'Other World'. The shaman's journey is undertaken with the intention of seeking information for the community or for a specific healing. Quite often, these journeys are also for the retrieval of lost souls or soul fragments lost to the individual.

In these other realities there are helpers; these are often animals, known as animal guides, and guides with more human appearances. The purpose of these guides is to provide assistance and lend support with healing. Usually shamans use a form of percussion, generally drumming or rattling to assist them in going into an ASC, allowing the free soul of the shaman to journey into these other worlds. Some traditions use a variation on the drum or rattle whereas other cultures use sticks or bells. In Australia, shamans will use a didgeridoo and, or click sticks, and the Sami people of Lapland use a monotonous chanting called 'joiking'. In the Keltic (ancient spelling of the modern

Celtic) tradition of the 'Path of Pollen', a method called tanging is used. The instrument is made from burnished copper, which resembles a small frying pan. The 'sound' is made by beating this 'drum' with two wooden sticks held together in one hand.

On examination of shamanic traditions around the world there are three common levels of journeying, known as worlds, which are consistently described. These are also often seen in artwork and paintings around the globe. These hidden worlds are known as the Lower World or Under World, the Middle World, and the Upper World. There are also numerous levels in the Upper and Lower worlds; all of which are outside of the concept of the space-time continuum. It is generally believed amongst shamans and some scientists that we live in an unlimited universe, limited only by our own mental limitations.

Every shaman has their own way of describing their journeying, and hence each interprets their journeys differently (*Heaven, 2003*). However, the commonality is in the way in which the shamans each journey to similar places in non-ordinary reality. The Lower World is reached by journeying through a tunnel that leads down into the earth. This is an earthy place, characterised by jungles, forests, oceans, lakes, caves and deserts. The beings that inhabit this world are the spirits of animals, plants, trees, and rocks, along with human spirits who are directly connected to the mysteries of the earth. My own principle guide here is a wise turtle called Maka (Earth Mother). Shamanic cultures believe that we are born with the spirit of at least two of these power animals, who have volunteered to keep us healthy emotionally and physically. They also protect us from harm. This is similar to the Christian belief of guardian angels.

The Upper World tends to be more etheric than the Lower World. It is very bright and often colourful; however, it can also be experienced as various shades of grey and even complete darkness. In this world the landscape is different, and there are often cities of crystal and clouds. There is a variety of different spirits that inhabit this world, often but not always, in human form. These typically were the gods and goddesses of each culture, religious figures, and ancestors who wished to help. My principle guide here is the Hindu God, Ganesh.

The Middle World is the hidden reality of the world in which we consciously live. In this world the shaman can move back and forth in 'time'. It is also the place where the shaman will journey to retrieve lost or stolen items. In this world the shaman is able to communicate with the spirits of all living things, the rocks, plants, trees, wind, water, fire, and earth. The Middle World is home to a variety of spirits often known as the 'hidden folk'. These are the fairies, elves, forest guardians and trolls of many of our myths and stories. These hidden folk remind us of the times when we were young and connected to these other realities before we closed the veils to these worlds.

Shamanic journeying is both an essential practice of shamanic work and an integral part of life in shamanic communities (*Bruce,* 2002). It is encouraged and discussed, often at length daily with the extended family and community, allowing it to develop into a way of life. This way of being creates other realms in which to learn and grow, other realities in which to play, rehearse, and other realms in which to live. In these cultures, these other realms are not thought of as any less real or useful than those we all experience in our daily lives. Journeying, therefore, is far more than personal fantasy. It is quite common practice for people to journey together, sharing these life experiences in much the same way as they share experiences in conscious reality.

Soul Loss and Retrieval

In many of the shamanic cultures it is believed that soul loss causes emotional and physical disease. In our culture we have doctors for our body and mind, but what happens when our spirit is ailing? In his groundbreaking work, Mircea Eliade (1951), describes a shaman as someone who makes a journey outside of the space-time continuum known to our conscious selves to retrieve whole or fragmented parts of our soul, to bring us back to health and wellness. Another way to look at this would be to view soul loss as a loss of our life force or vitality. This loss can take place when we suffer a trauma, have an accident, experience a strong emotional exchange with a loved one, the death of a loved one, separation, or divorce, or go through a time of other difficult personal circumstances. When we experience such traumas, we will often experience the temporary loss of some of our vital energy. This enables our body and consciousness to survive a severe traumatic event. The problems arise when the fragmented soul part does not return once the event is over. It may not feel it is able to come back, or even wants to come back due to the nature of the trauma.

Common symptoms of soul loss are feelings of not being 'all here', a sense of observing life rather than being fully engaged, a gap in memory, or chronic depression. Sandra Ingerman (1991) provides a useful checklist for indicators of soul loss as follows:

1. Do you ever have a difficult time staying 'present' in your body? Do you sometimes feel as if you're outside your body observing it as you would a movie?
2. Do you ever feel numb, apathetic, or detached?
3. Do you suffer from chronic depression?
4. Do you have problems with your immune system and trouble resisting illness?
5. Were you chronically ill as a child?
6. Do you have gaps in your memory of your life after five? Do you sense that you may have blacked out significant traumas in your life?
7. Do you struggle with addictions to, for example, alcohol, drugs, food, sex, or gambling?
8. Do you find yourself looking to external things to fill up an internal void or emptiness?

9. Have you had difficulty moving on with your life after a divorce or death of a loved one?
10. Do you suffer from multiple personality syndrome?

If we suffer from any of the above symptoms, it is likely that we are experiencing a soul loss, that vital parts of our energy are unavailable to us. Shamans believe that these soul fragments or parts exist in non-ordinary reality, and can be retrieved through shamanic journeying.

When a shaman embarks on a journey, he or she is being transported inwardly by a pulse or rhythmic sound, rather than outwardly around the face of the earth. This is not a physical journey, but one of entering an ASC in which they perceive realities outside of our normal awareness. Michael Harner (1980) coined the terminology, Shamanic State of Consciousness (SSC) for this ASC. The shaman's drum is the most common way for the shaman to enter ASC. As Jeanne Achterberg (1985) states, the drum, 'reigns as the most important means to enter other realities, and one of the most universal characteristics of shamanism.'

How drumming can evoke such changes in awareness is not fully understood. However, science is able to tell us that listening to a monotonous beat can cause the brain to produce brain waves in the alpha and theta ranges, rather than the beta waves of our eyes-open everyday consciousness. In his research called *The Mind Mirror*, Maxwell Cade (1979) states that theta waves are related to creativity, vivid imagery, and states of ecstasy. (Theta waves oscillate at 4-7 cycles per second.)

Native American people often refer to drumming as the 'heartbeat of the earth'. Whenever I hear the Native American drum at ceremonies I can feel it resonating through my body, as if my whole body is beating to the drum. This is supported by science, with the beat aligning itself with the electromagnetic resonance frequency of the earth. This has been measured at 7.5

cycles per second, equivalent to brain waves of the high theta, low alpha range (*Bentov,* 1979). It would therefore appear that drumming enables shamans to align their brain waves to those of the earth.

Shamans in many parts of the world also use other tools to assist them in retrieving lost souls. In Southeast Asia, the shaman will often use a box which contains a set of 'magical' objects, especially quartz crystals that are known as 'stones of light'. Shamans in other cultures will use objects called 'soul catchers', in British Columbia for example; this is a carved hollowed-out bone (Tsimshian shaman). Similarly, the Tungus shaman will use a noose to retrieve a lost soul (*Eliade,* 1951). Other shamans will have medicine pouches that contain sacred objects related to their power animal. For instance, a shaman who has a bear as his or her power animal may have a bear's claw, or if their power animal is an eagle, may have an eagle feather in their medicine pouches.

Power animals and guardian spirits are available to help the shamans carry out their work. They also believe that we each have at least one special guardian who protects and empowers us (*Harner, 1980*). An individual's guardian is also known as a power animal, and may be an eagle, a bear, a mouse, a lion, a woodpecker, or a dolphin. Each of these animals has its own area of expertise and power that it teaches us. A lion may teach us the power of stalking prey or protecting young, a woodpecker may teach us the power of chipping away at an obstacle, a dolphin may teach us to ride the waves of life and to connect to our spiritual self with ease. The shaman calls on his or her power animal to assist in the journey into non-ordinary reality. Part of the power animal's role is to assist the shaman in navigating these other realities. They may provide the shaman with specific information about what is wrong with someone, and what needs to be done to alleviate their illness, or specific steps they need to take in their lives.

A power animal can also provide assistance if the soul part is found in a place that is difficult to enter or leave, and can act as a scout to find the lost parts. A shaman may have several power animals, each providing their own particular support and advice. Likewise, some power animals may remain with the shaman for a lifetime, and others for a short period of time. The shaman can also be aided by helping spirits who come for an explicit purpose on a specific journey. For example, if the shaman needs to act quickly a horse may appear for the shaman to ride swiftly to a specific location, or a hawk may appear to take the shaman into the sky where he or she can see the whole picture.

My power animal, Maka, plays an interesting role. When I am working with clients, she will introduce me to the power animal of the client so that I can work directly with it to bring about healing. This gives me the benefit of a direct link to the skills and abilities that my client can tap into once our session is over, as well as using the very great skills and abilities of Maka, and my other guides.

When we enter ASC and then non-ordinary reality on a shamanic journey, the rules of our consensual reality are suspended. Plants talk, animals fly and our concepts of time and space are suspended. We may experience a sunrise and a sunset and yet have spent only thirty minutes in our ordinary time frame; we may also traverse great distances in a moment or two of outer world time.

Repeated journeys to other realities enable the shaman to develop a familiarity with certain territories. Once they have been to certain places like the cave of lost children a few times, they understand how best to retrieve souls from this place, it becomes a part of their territory. Just as many of us have special 'power' places in physical reality, a shaman has power places in non-ordinary reality where they can relax and reflect.

It was Eliade (1951) who classified the three major territories that a shaman journeys to; the Lower, Middle, and Upper worlds.

The names come from the direction that the shaman travels to get into these worlds. He describes these routes as taken via the Cosmic Tree, which is essential to the shaman. Its wood provides him or her with wood for their drum, and is the vehicle for reaching other worlds. Cosmologically, the World Tree rises at the centre of the earth, the place of the earth's umbilicus, and the upper braches make the connection with the cosmos.

At the beginning of his journey, the shaman clearly sets his intention; the purpose of the journey. He then travels into non-ordinary reality searching for the lost soul. Once it is found, it is his job to bring it back to ordinary reality. Traditionally this was achieved by cajoling, trickery, or some other means of catching the soul. However, the causes of soul loss are often less distinct in our modern world, with the trauma often caused by people who are themselves victims of some form of soul loss. So, modern day shamans tend to negotiate with the lost soul to bring it back. The lost soul is then able to choose to come back once it has learned that the original circumstances that caused it to leave have changed. From personal experience, I would describe this as a dialogue with the lost soul that enables it to reframe the original situation and release its previous fear and pain. The soul then agrees to return to the whole. (This is akin to a Parts Reframe in NLP.)

The key to journeying and shamanic healing lies in intention and trust. When undertaking soul retrieval it is imperative that the shaman's intent is absolutely clear. It is important that the shaman trusts his guides, and that the client trusts the shaman to undertake the soul retrieval on their behalf. These three elements combine to create the environment for healing. The shaman's role is to simply act as the vehicle through which healing occurs. A vehicle cannot drive itself; therefore, the shaman's responsibility is to ask the spirits for help, and to trust that it will be given.

The first step for the shaman is to meet the client and to understand the healing that is required. Once the shaman and client agree to do the healing, the shaman creates a sacred space to begin his or her work. Soul retrieval is a ceremony or ritual, usually carried out in the dark with the only light provided by a candle. The shaman lies down next to the client, and sets their intention as the drumming begins. The drumming allows him or her to set their intention and journey into non-ordinary reality by attaining an ASC. Here the shaman will meet their animal guide and or other guides, and journey to the place where the lost soul resides. He or she will then negotiate the return of the lost soul and bring it back to ordinary reality. The shaman will then return the soul to the client by blowing it into their heart space, and into the top of their head (crown chakra). This reintegration is felt as a sense of completeness, feeling lighter, and a sense of more energy.

Shamanic journeying is a powerful process and clients usually need some quiet time to allow the part to integrate fully. My approach is to leave the client alone for a while enabling them to become aware of their new feelings and for the integration process to complete. Very often they will want to discuss their experience as this too enables them to confirm the changes that have taken place.

Shapeshifting

Shapeshifting is something we all have the ability to do on a cellular level. We can learn how to shapeshift ourselves into a tree or a cat or any other form with which we have built an alliance. This may seem a little far-fetched but shapeshifting has been practised throughout shamanic cultures for eons. We can also shapeshift by bringing about fundamental changes in our attitudes and perceptions, and hence, our prosperity, health, appearance and personal relationships. In Paulo Coelho's book, *The Pilgrimage* (1999) he describes how he set about conquering the devil. His adversary took the form of a savage dog. The protagonist heard a spirit guide telling him that to survive he must turn himself into a dog. He was told that we must confront our opponents with the same weapons that are used against us. So Coelho, attacked the dog with his teeth and nails, he lunged at the dog's throat, and he apparently became so ferocious that he frightened a shepherd who was passing by. He shapeshifted and defeated the dog. This provides us with a great example of shapeshifting.

Shapeshifting takes off from a dream (*Perkins, 1997*), first a dream or vision must be created, and then the dreamer can transport him or herself into a new realm. Shamans have been known to shapeshift into bats, jaguars, and plants. Sometimes this can happen without conscious intent, enabling people to scale walls and undertake feats that they would be unable to accomplish in their ordinary reality. The shamans (and others) enter into an ASC and can then shapeshift themselves into another entity.

This happened to my former husband Robert, when he was in Sedona, Arizona on a spiritual retreat several years ago. He was with a group of people in the area around Bell Rock. They each found a place to sit and meditate, focusing on the energy of the land. Some time later, Robert became aware of people shouting, he opened his eyes and realised they were shouting at him. He found himself sat at the very top of a huge rock, which for him would have been a physical impossibility. As he started to descend, he clearly saw a gentle path down the rock, which he followed. No one else could see this pathway and were amazed at the ease of his descent. At that time he was very overweight and physically unfit; there was no way he could have ascended the apparently sheer rock face. Apparently this is a place that no one has been known to climb. He realised that he had shapeshifted into another creature capable of making the ascent and descent of that sheer rock.

According to Viejo Itza, a Mayan shaman (*Perkins, 1997*), we are mistaken if we think that we can shapeshift by simply taking on the appearance of something. In order to shapeshift, we have to become the other, but in fact, we do not become the other because we are the other all along. We and it are the same. To the modern mind, this may seem impossible, but according to shamanic thinking, it is simply a matter of energy. In our modern cultures, we tend to think in terms of organizations, giving our energy to changing corporations, or political parties, or institutions. When we want to change nature, her rivers, mountains, plants and animals, we use machines to overpower them. We convert parts of the earth into fuel in order to produce a type of energy that can be used as a technological hammer. However, shamanic cultures see energy from a simpler point of view.

Viejo Itza said that to create fire, in the western cultures we believe that we have to build a match or lighter factory; whereas the fire is within the wood and all we need to do is to rub two sticks together until they shapeshift into fire. Science, with our current limitations may not believe this, however many shamanic cultures believe that energy is everything and therefore everything is comprised of energy. Shapeshifting is simply a way of manipulating this energy, changing it from one form to another. The earth, the universe, us, animals, rocks, plants, buildings are all made up of energy. Whilst shamanic cultures understand this, in the Western world, we understand that a social relationship; that of husband and wife, father and daughter, mother and son, are intensely related. Most cannot see that this is true of ourselves with the whole of our physical and non-physical environment. We believe we can influence our relationship with our loved ones, or the direction of our business, and therefore we can. The shapeshifter believes that he or she can influence their relationship with the physical world, therefore they can.

It can be argued that this is an over simplification of life and that we need more than belief to achieve these shifts. However, if we were brought up in a culture where this was the norm, we would not think that this was anything out of the ordinary. In my research to date I have been unable to find any scientific evidence to support the process of shapeshifting. However, I have been able to find reported examples of shamans shapeshifting in a number of cultures.

This is best illustrated in a story told by John Perkins (*Shapeshifting, 1997*) when he met an Iranian man for dinner. The storyteller, Yamin, told him that each year he and his family would go into the desert for a week's holiday. One year when he was ten, his father promised him something special, the secret of the desert. The following morning before the sun had risen, Yamin and his father walked away from their tent. They trekked across the hot desert for hours until they reached a small oasis, where a Bedouin family lived amongst a clump of desert palms. They knew Yamin's father and welcomed them. After their evening meal, Yamin's father told him to go into the desert with the Bedouin man. They took two bedrolls and two goatskins filled with water and set off into the desert. They walked and walked, until Yamin had no idea where they were. Finally, they stopped to rest, lying out under the stars. Yamin fell asleep instantly.

When he awoke there was no sign of the Bedouin man, he jumped to his feet and shouted at the top of his lungs, he was terrified. He began to wander around, searching for a clue. He found nothing, no tracks, just lots of sand. He panicked and began running. He ran until he fell onto the sand sobbing and afraid, realising that he had no idea where he was, or where he was going. For the first time in his young life he confronted death. He felt completely helpless in this foreign environment. He pleaded with Allah, and nothing happened, so he buried himself into the sand for comfort. When he eventually opened his eyes he spotted some tracks, they were his own, excited, he followed them until he saw that they took him to a circle where he sat down. He closed his eyes and released his fear, opening himself to the desert. It was then that he heard a voice. The voice told him that the desert is kind once you accept it, once you learn to be a part of it. He opened his eyes and standing over him was the Bedouin man. He had been there all along, wrapped in his bedroll, covered in sand. He had never let Yamin out of his sight. The Bedouin had 'shapeshifted' into the sand.

Whilst it could be argued that this story is anecdotal and has no proof, and could even be metaphorical, I have included it as an example of the beliefs and therefore the reality of different peoples of this world. Arguably, if we take the perspective that shapeshifting is yet to be proven, I would ask, then why is it accepted as an integral part of indigenous cultures around the world?

Many shamanic cultures believe that the biggest global shapeshift in recent times has been the most disastrous in human history. This was the shift away from being in balance with nature into the survival of the fittest, a very ego centric concept. There is a great deal of discussion today about pollution and the depletion of the world's resources moving us towards a point of no return in the viability of our world and those who populate it. The shaman that I worked with in the Andes described this as the world slowly shapeshifting from a place of balance and harmony with nature, to one of corporate domination and pollution. It is as if money and an obsession with collecting 'stuff' have almost become sacred.

A number of the shamans I have spoken to view Christ as a great shaman and shapeshifter. They say that he came to help humanity but realized that the only way we would learn about this imbalance was through direct experience. We need to suffer all the luxury, all the materialism, and economic progress, in order to understand what we really desire. They believe that Christ lit a fire that has stayed ignited in our hearts and that nothing has been able to squash this. They also believe that we will shapeshift again, and that the Revolution in the USA was almost such a shapeshift.

Sadly, a few of the younger shamans I have met in recent times are being greatly influenced by the lifestyle of the Western World, and are adopting a style of materialism. I met one such 'shaman' in Peru in the spring of 2008; his focus was on what he could gain materially and monetarily. The result was that his ceremonies lacked the authenticity of many of the others I have worked with, and the results reflected this.

Several of the Shamans I have spoken to (Don Ramon, Don Alberto, Maestro Juan) believe that until we overcome our fear of shapeshifting we will never be able to shapeshift ourselves, or our cultures. If we feel that a tree is inferior to us, how can we overcome any fear of becoming one? Some shapeshifters never return to their original form, as they choose not to. However, whilst they believe that we fail to accept that a being, a tree, or a fish is every bit as good, if not better, than being a human, then we should stick to shapeshifting our institutions and organisations.

In order to effectively shapeshift we must understand the importance of our dream about how we want life to be, or the form we wish to shapeshift into. To shapeshift, it is important to distinguish between a dream and a fantasy, to be able to separate one from the other. This is an integral part of clarifying intent. Dreams are things we want to turn into reality, and fantasies are not, they are simply fantasies. When these two become muddled, fantasies come true because we believe that they are dreams.

Put very simply, to shapeshift we must allow our energy to slip into the energy of the tree, or as in the story of the Bedouin, slip into the energy of the desert. In shamanic cultures, death is also seen simply as a shapeshift from this reality to another, and one we all learn to do. We just pass on and take on a new form. This takes away all the angst that people of the modern world associate with their own death and that of their loved ones.

Guided visualisations are a modern-day way of assisting

people into shapeshifting. CDs and tapes of these guided journeys enable people to attain health and well-being with repeated use. I have personally used these to help people become healthier, to release excess weight, to overcome problems, to have more energy amongst others. By following the guidance on the tapes, people are able to relax, set their intention and dream, creating a shapeshift and a new personal reality.

Another example of shifting out of something is a modification of a traditional fire ceremony of the Maya, living in the Guatemalan highlands. A doll is made out of natural flammable materials such as grasses, leaves, twigs and flowers. This doll becomes the representation of the person who makes it. Permission is asked of all the materials before they are taken and used. Whilst constructing the doll, the maker blows the energy or the spirit of the thing to be released into the doll; in other words, they are focusing on shifting some aspect of their life. It can be an emotion, an addiction, a job, a physical illness, or a relationship. The person then spends some time meditating with the doll, focusing on the desired shift. A fire ceremony is then held and the doll is presented to the fire, taking away the dis-ease and releasing it to Mother Earth, who recycles the energy.

There are many recorded examples of shamans shapeshifting dis-ease into visible intrusions that can be removed from the patient, or of shamans shapeshifting into other creatures, such as bats swooping through a sick person drinking up fluids that threaten their lives, and then regurgitating them.

Most of us shapeshift our lives and health on a daily basis without any conscious awareness; by entering ASC with clear intent, we can shapeshift our lives in small ways to create health and well-being.

The Path of Pollen

The Path of Pollen is an ancient Keltic, shamanistic practice which has continued out of the conscious awareness of most people for centuries. Keltic is the old spelling of the more modern word Celtic, and was the name given to many of the tribes of Northern Europe during pre-medieval times. The Path of Pollen is even more ancient than this, as we find examples of Bee Shamanism throughout the world, each growing from very ancient and parallel roots.

Throughout history, there is no other species of animal that has inspired people in so many ways, as has the honeybee. No creature has had more literature devoted to it from the time of Aristotle to the present day. For thousands of years, men and women have worked alongside the bee, and throughout this time we have come to view this little creature with a great deal of respect. The bee is, therefore, often used to represent purity, integrity, and industry, along with other perceived virtues. I recall seeing images of bees in the hieroglyphs in the ancient healing temples of Egypt. The bee has been a part of our lives, as long as we have had lives. The bee is also the foundation of life here on earth. Without bees to pollinate plants and trees, there would be little, if any food on this planet. The bees fertilise the plants, grasses, and trees, animals eat the plants, and we eat the animals and the plants. Sadly, bees are now disappearing in their millions, due to forced feeding and a variety of diseases. This has to raise the question, where will life on earth be if we no longer have healthy bee populations?

In his illuminating book, *The Shamanic Way of the Bee* (2004), Simon Buxton talks about the many cultures around the world that practise 'bee mastery'. Some suggest that this book was written as a work of semi- fiction however, if we choose to reflect on this it becomes apparent that most cultures around the world acknowledge the bee as a fundamental pillar of life on earth. Without the bee many of our plants would not be pollinated and therefore we would not have as many diverse plants and hence, food. I am therefore including this section for completeness in my review of information available about shamanism and shamanic practices.

Australian Aborigines would wait at a water hole for bees to come and collect water. They would then flick a special weed that exudes a sticky gum to stick a piece of feather fluff onto the bee's back. This would weigh it down so that it could be followed and the hive located, enabling them to collect and eat the sweet honey. The bee shamans of the Kayapo people in Brazil have great skill in identifying different stingless bees, and locating their nests. The bees would always leave behind honey 'for Bep-kororoti, the great bee shaman who was taken into the sky in a flash of lightening'. The first initiation into the Path of Pollen is a twenty-three day process, during which the initiate drinks mead (a drink brewed from honey), known as a metheglin or medicine. The ancient Greeks called it ambrosia, the drink of the gods. In combination with the power and communion with the hive, it is said to have magical and sacred properties.

Allegedly, the Path of Pollen holds information and methodology that has been held in trust for millennia. It is publicly, and yet discretely used when needed for healing and to deepen communion with the hidden universe. The bee sting, known as the Sacramental Venom, or the Secret Fire, is a powerful and mystical substance, which can transmute illness into wellness. According to Buxton (2004), Hippocrates, the father of modern medicine was an initiate in the usage of Sacramental Venom. It is also thought by some scholars that those who hold a deeper communion with the hive are the original acupuncturists, using the bee sting in the same way as an acupuncturist uses their needles.

Full initiation into the Path of Pollen is by invitation and consists of a gruelling initiation, using the Sacramental Venom. Ambiguous behaviour is used to create an ASC, where the usual ordinary consciousness can no longer operate, and a new state of awareness is attained. This state is deepened with tanging (the use of a small metal drum known as a quoit), putting the shaman into a true ASC. This is the same as the Shamanic State of Consciousness seen in other shamanic cultures. In this state, the bee shaman does his work. The initiate is then deliberately stung on both sides of the neck, to receive the Sacramental Venom. This process is repeated on the crown of the head, known as the dream wheel, and then in the place midway between the eyebrows. The result is a retching and violent purge similar to that induced by ayahuasca, the teacher plant, followed by a loss of consciousness. The initiate then spends twenty-three days in a hexagonal cocoon, an oneiricell, (from the Greek word oneiros, to dream). They drift in and out of consciousness, feeding only on a diet of pollen and honey, and experiencing a dying of the old self and a rebirth of the new.

The day of a bee shaman starts with rising at dawn and spending about forty-five minutes performing the lemniscatic walk (walking the shape of the sign of infinity). This is the dance that bees do when they come back from foraging to tell the hive where the best nectar is. The walk is believed to give the shaman access to infinite knowledge and vitality. They then eat some pollen (golden coins), and fruit, all meals are eaten mindfully in silence.

Bee shamans work with animals and people who desire healing. Tanging and singing are used to enable the shaman to enter an ASC to journey to other realities to obtain information for the client from outside of our conscious space-time continuum. The shaman also imbibes bee venom during the day, as it is believed to assist the shaman in remaining healthy. It is also used as an integral part of any healing for conditions as diverse as arthritis and shingles.

In this shamanic tradition, men and women shamans have different and distinct roles, as in the hive. The Bee Mistress and her female apprentices are called, the Melissae. The Melissae are the mysterious veiled women of the hive, their two central powers are the knowledge of destiny and the ability to inspire. Men are guests of the bee tradition, and the Melissae are the hosts. Bee society represents the zenith of the female potency of nature, whereas the men are simply drones. The basics of masculinity and femininity have not been changed in a thousand years. According to bee tradition, the female consistently does more reproductive work, and the male is in some ways a parasite on his partner. However, in the larger scheme of life both the Bee Master and the Bee Mistress are distinct, and of equal importance, as they maintain balance and equilibrium within their community.

Plant Medicine

Plants have been an integral part of the lives of human beings throughout our evolution. They not only provide us with food and medicine, but they are also a great source of beauty and fragrance. Their natural healing and spiritual qualities provide us with a gateway to the Great Mystery, which our Celtic ancestors called 'the visible face of spirit'. In our modern frenetic world we view a weekend in the country or by the ocean as a treat, something we do not have time for in our normal everyday busy lives. Yet, Nature herself has the ability to relax, refresh, or excite us, simply by spending time with her. I know that if I am feeling out of balance, a simple walk in the fresh air of the countryside or a quiet rest in a beautiful garden makes me feel so much better and balance is restored.

Flowers play an important part in our lives, whether we are consciously aware of it or not. We give flowers to a friend who may be feeling unwell; they also play a part in our weddings, funerals and birthdays. They may be a part of new beginnings, the first, 'I love you', and they are there at the end after death. However, in our modern materialistic world we have forgotten the mythical and spiritual connections we have with Nature. We simply give flowers at key times in people's lives, 'because that is what is done' without a deeper understanding of our forebears.

(Heaven, and Charing, 2006).

Likewise, we treat our diseases with laboratory manufactured synthetic drugs, many of which are synthetic derivatives of the plants used by rainforest shamans to cure diseases naturally. This is the result of us no longer seeing ourselves as part of nature, but as 'masters' of nature.

An old shaman from the Salascan tribe, on the eastern slopes of the Andes, has suggested that psychotropic plants should be used akin to a corkscrew to open a hole in the top of our heads, giving us access to the wider consciousness through ASCs. He is also of the view that once we allow all the knowledge to flow in, it is no longer necessary to use psychotropic plants *(Perkins, 1994).*

I have had the pleasure and honour of meeting several shamans who believe that all knowledge is within us, and that the appropriate use of psychotropic drugs alters our consciousness by simply opening our heads so that we can listen to the dreams, and hence, access different levels of consciousness.

Plant shamans are those who specialise in the use of plants for healing and bringing balance to people and situations. They work with a number of visionary teacher plants, each of which has a spirit maestro to help them connect with the living and other worlds. This is the domain of the sacred hallucinogens. To the majority in the Western world this simply means these plants can produce hallucinations and 'trips'. However, for the shaman we are all dreaming or hallucinating, and the taking of sacred plants simply enables us to access other dimensions of reality to assist in the healing process.

According to these shamans, our modern cities and ways of being in the west are based on our 'dreams'. We have dreamed ourselves into this reality. As mentioned earlier, they say this dream is one of separation and disconnection from the flow of life, creating competition, conflict, and challenge as our norms. The fact that life doesn't need to be this way and that we could create a different dream, one based on a more connected model, would suggest to a shaman that we are going through a mass hallucinatory experience.

Sacred hallucinogens offer us a means of breaking out of this living trance into an expansive, freeing, rich universe full of infinite possibilities for other realities and futures. For the majority of people this is a terrifying thought. In a culture where ego is dominant, the thought of side stepping the ego and seeing reality in a new way can shake the very foundation of our belief systems. However in truth, rather than leading us away from ourselves and out of balance as with many of the chemical hallucinogens such as LSD, these plants help us to go deeper inside of ourselves to a place of greater balance through genuine self awareness (*McKenna, 1992*).

The power of these visionary plants requires that they be taken as an integral part of a spiritual ritual, with a clear intention or purpose. The word hallucination implies a primarily visual experience, however for the shaman it is much more than that. Visions do come, but these teacher plants also bring with them an intense sense of oneness with the world, deep and profound insights, and a merging with the field of creative consciousness. In essence the teacher plants offer the shaman a way into the hidden realms of human consciousness and the spiritual intelligence of a living planet.

Ayahuasca

One of the most potent and well-known sacred hallucinogens is ayahuasca, otherwise known as 'the vine of the soul'. This brew is known as ayahuasca in Ecuador and Peru, is also known as yage in Columbia and caape in Brazil. It is used in healing from North Western Columbia to the lowlands of Bolivia, and to the east and west of the Andes. The Ashaninca people of the Upper Amazon (*Narby, 1998*) are said to work their magic through direct communication with cellular DNA, which is the building block of planetary life. By taking ayahuasca in ceremony they alter their consciousness to go beyond nature to the stuff from which all of nature and all things are made, merging with the 'global network of DNA based life'.

Many people report that when they take ayahuasca they experience visions of serpents, often two intertwined. It was the similarities of these visions, the ayahuasca vine itself and DNA, that led Narby (1998) to suggest that through attaining ASCs, shamans are able to communicate directly with the information stored in DNA. Narby further studied the characteristics of DNA and discovered that it emits electromagnetic waves that correspond to the narrow band of visible light, the equivalent to the intensity of a candle at a distance of ten kilometres. It also had a surprisingly high degree of coherence, comparable to a laser. Narby speculates that this may be the waveform of consciousness itself, he further speculates that plant medicines such as ayahuasca provide the means of making this visible by their ability to alter our states of consciousness.

Ayahuasca is made from the ayahuasca vine (Banisteriopsis Caapi), combined with the leaf of the chacruna plant (Psychotria Viridis). In Quechua, aya means, 'spirit', ancestor or dead person; Huasca means, vine or rope. Therefore, this can be loosely translated to mean, 'vine of the dead soul' or 'spirit of the universe'. It is even more interesting that each plant on its own is inert. Chacruna, contains tryptamines, amino acids which if ingested alone are rendered inactive by our body's own enzymes, and the ayahuasca vine has monoamine oxidase (MAO) inhibitors, in the form of harmine compounds. When combined, the two complement each other and create a psychoactive compound. This compound has the identical chemical make-up to the organic tryptamines in our body. It can therefore travel throughout our body to the synaptic receptor sites, and slowly release tryptamines into our bodies, creating a powerful visionary experience. Western science 'discovered' the mechanism of MAO inhibitors in the 1950s, (*Eliade, 1950*) whereas shamans have known of this by 'listening' to the plants for centuries.

Narby further describes the ASCs attained by taking ayahuasca as a series of fast moving visions, creating a kaleidoscope of geometric images. These then change into brightly coloured masks, serpents, and shapeshifting faces, and sometimes cartoons. In *Plant Spirit Shamanism (2006)*, co-authored by Ross Heaven and Howard Charing, they describe an experience Howard had as one of feeling like his brain had been re-patterned and his consciousness altered, enabling him to enter into dialogue with the deeper spirit of ayahuasca and its spiritual intelligence. He believes that by going beyond the visions, and having direct communication with the ayahuasca spirit, information of great value is revealed for all types of healing. For example, the ayahuasca spirit may tell the shaman what is wrong with his patient, which medications to prescribe or what has caused the illness in the first place. Throughout my research in this area, numerous shamans are quoted as saying that they are able to access the intelligence that permeates the universe through ingesting ayahuasca, and that this is where they are able to receive gifts of insight and self-awareness.

Don Alberto, an Amazonian shaman that ran an ayahuasca healing ceremony at my home, tells us that ayahuasca is a teacher plant that helps us to access our great inner knowledge by removing the obstacles our everyday conscious constructs in our minds. In preparing for the ceremony, he told us that the spirit of ayahuasca opens our mind to that which cannot be seen in normal consciousness. For example by altering our consciousness in this way, we may see a tree that has its own world and spirit, and by experiencing this, we can see and accept the mystery of it all. The set-up for the ceremony was very beautiful with Don Alberto chanting icaros (sacred songs) and calling in the spirits.

I had made the decision to undertake the ceremony after some very serious thought. As a young college student, I had never been drawn to the hallucinogenic sessions of my fellow students, taking the view that such activities were potentially dangerous. However, after studying shamanism, meeting Don Alberto, and appreciating the sacredness of the whole experience, I felt it was important that I participate in at least one ayahuasca healing ceremony.

A small group of about five of us sat in the dark under the apple trees in our orchard as Don Alberto started to chant and invoke the spirits to assist us. We sat in a small circle in our sleeping bags, receptacles at hand for vomiting, and waited. I had a small glass of the orange liquid, which tasted a little sour, and listened to the chanting. We were offered more, but I declined thinking one small glass would be sufficient. My mind drifted gently as I listened to the sound of Don Alberto's voice and then the sky started to turn wonderful shades of deep peach and orange, 'Oh, I am having a vision,' I thought, and then I realised the sun was rising. I looked around at our little group huddled in our sleeping bags and wondered if anyone had experienced an ASC. None of us had seen anything other than the sun rising, and I have to say we were disappointed. Maybe it was because the shaman had watered down the ayahuasca for bringing it to Europe, or maybe there was something energetic going on within the group. Suffice to say that this clearly was not the time or the place for us to experience the power of the vine of the soul. However, I was not discouraged by the experience and feel that it took away any residual fear I had about using sacred hallucinogenic plants for healing. This experience also reinforced for me the importance of undertaking this work in a sacred way with an experienced shaman rather than the casual recreational use of drugs in our culture.

Another powerful and respected elder of the ayahuasca tradition, Guillermo Arvela, told a group on a recent visit to the

Amazon that ayahuasca organises our emotions and calms the nerves. It enables people who are depressed to discover their own solutions, recover their self-esteem, and access their spiritual sides. He also told them that when people are out of balance they only recognise their physical side and ignore their spiritual self. This is due to cultural beliefs and the way in which we are educated, that separates us from reality and keeps us in one type of consciousness, that of science, logic, and religion. This results in separation from 'all that is'; the universal consciousness.

Ayahuasca is a healer and teacher, so by taking it in a ceremonial we expand our consciousness, regaining our power and lucidity. Past traumas can be healed and hurts resolved, this is said to be the purpose of ayahuasca. It is evident from all the people I have spoken to, and my personal experiences with the vine in Peru in 2008 that ayahuasca has a great ability to heal. This healing is facilitated by a seemingly paradigm shift in our consciousness. To my mind, this starts with the intention at the very outset of the healing process, and hence the physical making of the medicine.

Shamans from many different tribes and cultures believe that plants have angelic spirits. However, they are also said to have human emotions such as vengefulness and wrath. It is because of this aspect of the plant that the medicine has to be prepared with great care and respect to prevent the plant spirit from becoming vengeful. My personal perspective is that it is the intention and attention of the process that is important. By focusing on the purpose of the healing session, and placing attention on the process of preparing the plant for this session, we are aligning our energy and consciousness. Opening our minds (expanding our consciousness) and remaining focused on the outcome is fundamentally important to any healing process. Another way to look at this is to say that the process requires love and attention. If the energy in this preparation phase is one of love then this provides a clear channel for the healing to take place, without the clutter of extraneous thoughts and distractions.

Ayahuasca takes twelve hours of careful preparation. According to some of the research I have undertaken, the shaman follows a special diet and carefully tends the fire throughout the process. Only designated helpers or trainee shaman are allowed to assist, and they too should follow the same diet and keep their focus on working with the plants to create a healing, and directing healing energy into the brew. The patient is never allowed to participate in this part of the process.

My experience in Peru was somewhat contrary to this as everyone in the group participated in preparing the ayahuasca and arguably we were both patients and 'trainee' shamans. However, the whole process was conducted as an integral part of the ceremony. We each selected a part of the vine that had previously been collected by Don Enrique, the Shaman, to prepare and add to the bubbling brew heated over a fire in the open. We were told to focus on our intention and gently beat the vine to break through the toughened outer layer to enable the chemicals to be released into the brew more easily. We did this in turn, and said a prayer as we added our 'stick' into the pot. When we had completed this, Enrique sang his icaros, remaining with the pot until the medicine was ready later that evening.

The icaros change the shaman's consciousness by focusing his or her energy into the brew, and they continue to sing throughout the ceremonial ingestion. The shaman will also sing their icaros into the energy field of the person to be healed to assist them in changing their consciousness, enabling the healing to take place. Each icaro is seen as an energetic force infused with positive or healing intent. The songs are said to be given, or transmitted to the shaman, by the spirit of the plant allies with whom he has a relationship. Usually the longer the shaman has had a relationship with the plant allies the more icaros he or she has.

Tobacco is deemed as one of the most sacred plants in the Amazon, and the 'icaro de tabaco' (tobacco song) is one of the most sacred songs of the plant shaman. Nature is regarded as a shaman's greatest teacher and authority, so most power songs come directly from nature. However, occasionally a song is passed from shaman to apprentice, so some songs are many centuries old.

Urban ayahuasca healing sessions are emerging in cities like Iquitos in Peru. Marlene Dobkin de Rios *(1990)* reports that slum-dwelling people of the city consult a Mestizo shaman (mixed blood), who uses ayahuasca. These shamans are known as ayahuasqueros.

The Cactus of Vision – San Pedro

The San Pedro cactus (Trichocereus Panchanoi) is found in Northern Peru. It is known as the cactus of vision because it is known to expand the awareness of those who ingest it in sacred ceremonies. It grows specifically on the dry eastern slopes of the Andean mountains, at around 2,000 to 3,000 meters. It grows very tall, reaching in excess of six meters. Traditionally, it has been grown in the medicine gardens of the shaman for at least 3000 years. The earliest depiction of this sacred cactus (*Evans Schultes, & Hoffman, 1992*) is seen in a carving believed to be dated around 1300 BCE. The carving, from the Chavin culture, shows a mythical being holding a San Pedro cactus and can be seen in the temple at Chavin de Huantar in the northern Peruvian highlands. It can also be seen in the later iconography of the Mochina culture, around 500 CE.

A story is told that the cactus is named after St Peter who allegedly used its magical powers to find the keys to heaven, to enable people to share paradise. The cactus was given his name in respect of his Promethean intervention on behalf of mortal men. However, the missionaries believed that San Pedro enabled the natives to speak with the devil. As might be imagined, the shaman's perspective is very different. Juan Navarro, a maestro of the San Pedro tradition, describes the effects as a dreamy state leading to a vision, a clearing of all faculties and a sense of tranquillity. I worked with Juan Navarmo when in Peru in the spring of 2008. He says that this visual force incorporates all senses, including the sixth sense, a telepathic sense of being transported across time and matter, as if thoughts are removed to a distant dimension.

San Pedro is literally considered to be the maestro of maestros, opening a portal between the visible and invisible worlds. It is known in Quechua as *punka*, which means doorway. Similarly, as with ayahuasca, healing with San Pedro is an intricate sequence of processes. It starts with an invocation, followed by diagnosis, divination and healing with natural power objects such as stones, shells, and crystals, known as *Artes*. The artes are laid out on a mesa, an altar, usually a cloth, in front of the shaman. He then ingests the San Pedro to expand his consciousness and to facilitate a healing.

As described earlier, my experience of San Pedro was the most powerful healing experience I have had with plant medicine. When I evaluate this along with my other experiences, it suggests to me that the combination of the natural power of the plant combined with the integrity, knowledge and experience of the Shaman were the important components to this effectiveness.

Dr John Lilly (*1995*), suggests in his research that the key to these healings seems to be that many of the sacred hallucinogens contain neurotransmitters that occur naturally in the human body, which can be enhanced with the development of specific practices. In his research into floatation tanks and ASCs, Lilly discovered that when the mind is deprived of external stimuli it opens to unusual sensations and spiritual effects, such as waking visions, lucid dreaming, and some out of body experiences.

Peyote

This sacred hallucinogen is thought to have been in use for several thousand years before Europeans discovered the

Americas. Remains found in dry caves and rock shelters in Texas, suggest the ceremonial use of peyote for three millennia *(Bear, Sun, 1987)*. Scientific evaluation of the plant has demonstrated antibiotic activity more potent than penicillin plus other medical and psychological benefits *(Mount, 1993)*. The Incas are said to have used peyote in brain surgery. Later, it developed into a sacrament for use in religious ceremonies amongst the people living along the Rio Grande.

One of the best-known examples of the medicinal use of peyote is its use in childbirth, which links back to the stories of its origin. It continues to be used as an herb amongst unlicensed spiritual midwives who learned its use from a number of different Native American traditions. Their testimonies and experiences describe joyful and even ecstatic births rather than the arduous experience of many western women. According to Guy Mount in his book, *The Peyote Book, A Study of Native Medicine (1993),* several tribes in Mexico and the United States tell a story like this:

> *A woman is lost in the desert. She is in labour, starving, and afraid. 'Something' tells her to eat peyote. Then she delivers the child easily. Her hunger is gone and her breasts are full of milk. Her strength and sense of direction return. She carries the new baby and a basket of peyote back to the people.*

There are numerous variations on this story from several of the Mexican Indian tribes, along with the Apaches, Tonkawas, Kiowa and Comanches.

Peyote is known throughout the Native American cultures as the 'Good Medicine'. It is a small cactus found in abundance where the desert is undisturbed. Plants grow in the desert along the Rio Grande in southern Texas and into Mexico, where people have gathered the buttons for thousands of years. From here, the ancient traders took it to the tribes in the north. It used to be quite abundant in Texas until modern dry cattle ranching and the development of the Texan oil wells spoilt the desert. Ranchers plant buffalo grass and create huge pastures, resulting in the peyote disappearing at a rate of 20 acres per hour where the ploughing machines operate (*Mount, 1993*). It is therefore very important that peyote is harvested carefully to ensure it survives in these areas. Until 1972 it was legal to cultivate and sell peyote, however, as a part of President Nixon's fight against drugs this became illegal.

Peyote is seen as a sacred herb, a healer and teacher plant that guides the body to health and the mind to spiritual awareness. When collecting peyote it is important to leave the roots so that new crown can grow, producing new buttons the following season. The buttons contain a cottony substance which has to be removed; the buttons can then be made into tea or chewed completely. They apparently taste like strong bitter chocolate (*Schultes, 1972*).

Peyote is at the heart of the Native American Church, and is known as the holy herb. This church unites people from all tribes and religions; whilst they may not speak the same language they understand each other spiritually. Peyote power is 'the knowledge of God through peyote' (*Erdoes, 1996*). It is used as a holy sacrament of the church, which peyote roadmen say is as old as the earth. The word peyote comes from the Uto Aztecan *peyotly*, this means caterpillar, because the peyote cactus is fuzzy like a caterpillar.

The Native American Church rituals are beautiful; a man called Quanah Parker (*Zemlicka, & Knudson, 2004*) originally founded them. His ritual became known as the crossfire ceremony as a Bible was used in it, and cornhusk cigarettes smoked. Later non Christian Indians founded the moon fire ceremony. They did not have the Bible and used the sacred pipe rather than cornhusk cigarettes. Whether these meetings take place in a building or a tipi, the set-up is the same. There are nuances that are different between a moon fire and a crossfire meeting, and also between a Lakota and Navajo meeting, but they are essentially the same. All the things that are used at a meeting – the drum, staff, gourd, and fan – are handled in a specific manner.

The road chief, who leads people on the road of life, sits on the west, opposite the entrance (*Erdoes, 1996*). To the right of the road chief sits the drummer, and to his left, the cedar man, who uses cedar as incense throughout the meeting. The fireman sits at the east by the door, his job is to tend the fire and act as doorkeeper. Close to him, sits the water carrier, who is always a woman (usually the wife or daughter of the road chief). The road chief has his holy objects, a staff, gourd, feather fan, eagle bone whistle, and in front of him is an altar cloth. Some members also bring their own sacred objects. If the sacred pipe is used it has a special stand in front of the road chief. In front of the pipe rest is a half moon altar made of sand on which 'Grandfather Peyote' is placed. Then there is the sacred fire and the sacred food, a pail of water, corn, meat, and chokecherries, all representing sacred aspects of life.

The drum represents the Indian's heartbeat; it contains seven pebbles representing the seven sacraments, or seven camp circles of the Lakota nation. The drumstick represents the stick the government uses to beat the Indian.

The staff is the staff of authority or unity. Thoughts and prayers travel up the staff, and the vision from above travels down to the participants, this is the Grandfather peyote vision.

The gourd is a rattle and represents the Indian's head; it is a shelter for thoughts and minds. Each part of the ritual is an important step in achieving ASC and all have a specific purpose, usually a healing for someone. The ceremonies themselves last about twelve hours. Each peyote roadman (ceremonial leader) has his own version of how to conduct ceremony. However, every ceremony will finish with a morning prayer and everyone shares a meal together. Many people report miraculous healings taking place at these ceremonies.

Carl Hamamerschlag M.D. (1988) describes his experiences with the peyote church as all encompassing. He describes how he sings Jewish songs and prayers at the ceremonies, and wears his father's prayer shawl, the one he wore at his bar mitzvah in Germany. Carl says his Indian friends have told him that it does not matter which language we use because there are always at least two people who understand, you and your creator. He says, 'the more you work with your mind, the more you realise you cannot know it. The more you seek to reach your spirit, the more you realise that you must enter some altered state of consciousness to burst free of the conventional limitations of flesh and rationality. This is what the peyote church is all about.'

The peyote plant (Lophophora williamsii) like its relative, ayahuasca, contains alkaloids that are proven to be healing agents (*Schultes, 1972*). It contains more than thirty alkaloids and their amine derivatives. Each one of these is bio dynamically active, however, their effects are not yet well understood. Phenyletylamine mescaline is the vision-inducing alkaloid and others are reported to be responsible for the tactile and auditory hallucinations. There are some very real differences between peyote hallucinations and those of mescaline. With peyote, it is the whole of the button that is ingested with the whole of its alkaloid content, whereas mescaline contains just one alkaloid, without the physiological interaction of the others that are present in the whole plant.

Peyote is an effective antibiotic (*Dorrance, 1975 & Walkington, 1960*) against many strains of bacteria, especially some strains that are resistant to penicillin. It is also an antiseptic, cleaning open cuts and wounds, encouraging a strong flexible scab that draws the skin together and seals it more effectively than stitches. It is proven to cure alcoholism and drug addictions, and relieves distress and acute depression (soul loss). Peyote is non toxic and spiritually nourishing as well as a great home remedy for a number of common ailments such as arthritis, rheumatism, pleurisy, colds and flu, hearing disorders and childbirth, to name a few.

I have discovered one account where the use of peyote in rituals was deemed to cause conflict, and has subsequently been proscribed (*Sun Bear, 1987*). Apparently, the Apaches on the Mescalero used peyote in their ceremonial healings between 1870 and 1910, however; it was abandoned because of the antagonism and violence that ensued. Traditionally, only the shaman would imbibe the hallucinogen for a sacred healing ritual, however, in peyote ceremonies all participants partake. Apparently, this caused rivalry between participants as people competed for authority, vying for supremacy of power, and status. The physiopsychological effects of the peyote reduced the repression of long-seated hostilities, leading to bloodshed. So, it was decided to ban the use of peyote on the reservation.

Sacred Mushrooms

Munn studied the use of psychotropic mushrooms, (Psilocybe Mexicana) in Hauntla de Jumenez (*Harner, 1973*). They contain the alkaloids, psilocybine and psilocine, which pass quickly through the system and are excreted in urine. The shamans who ingest these mushrooms during healing ceremonies understand this and will drink their urine to extend the duration of their hallucinations, or offer it to other participants as a special treat.

The Mazatec people of Oaxaca in Mexico will only eat their sacred mushrooms (Psilocybe Mexicana Heim) at night. They believe that if they are eaten during the daylight, the person eating them will go mad. They are also eaten in pairs, representing man and woman, the dual principles of creation. The Mazatec say that the mushrooms speak through the shaman as he performs his healing. The psychedelic experience is inseparably associated with the curing of an illness. This is because illness is not seen as physical in origin, but as mental or ethical. Hence, these mushrooms are only eaten when someone needs a healing.

The Use of Hallucinogens in Medieval Europe

It appears to be a little-known fact that the use of hallucinogens in Europe for healing was once commonplace. This is principally because such activities were driven underground by the Inquisition, as they were deemed as heretical. It is only in recent years that the use of botanicals in ancient European rituals has become known.

The most important group of plants used in sacred rituals across the world are the Solanaceae. This is the potato family and includes; the potato, tomato, chilli peppers, tobacco, and the genus Datura, all of which are hallucinogenic, (*Grob*, *2002*). Datura has been used since ancient times in shamanism in Europe, Asia, Africa, and the American continent. Other hallucinogens in the potato family closely resembling Datura in their effects are: mandrake (Mandragonia), now of Harry Potter fame, henblane (Hyoscyamus) and belladonna or deadly nightshade (Atrope belladonna). They are found throughout both temperate and tropical climates and all continents. Each of these plants contains varying amounts of atropine and other related alkaloids, all of which are hallucinogenic in nature. They can be extremely dangerous in their mental and physical effects and toxicity, which can result in death.

Children in our culture are taught that witches fly through the air on broomsticks. It is actually symbolic of a very serious and central aspect of ancient European witchcraft involving solanaceae hallucinogenic plants. European witches rubbed their bodies with hallucinogenic ointments made from plants such as Atrope belladonna, mandragonia and henblane. The hallucinogenic properties were then absorbed through the skin. This is the journey, represented by witches on their broomsticks, where the witch travels to meet with the spirits to invoke a healing.

Combining Anthropology with Biology

In his groundbreaking work in the late 1990s, the Swiss anthropologist, Jeremy Narby (2006), combines the science of biology with his direct anthropological experience. He is able to combine the hitherto subjective and anecdotal study of shamanism with science. His research demonstrates to his satisfaction that in their visions, shamans shift their consciousness to the molecular level. Here, they have access to information related to DNA, which they call 'animate essences' or 'spirits'. At this level, shamans are able to see the double helixes, twisted ladders, and chromosome shapes. He claims that this is how for millennia, shamanic cultures have known that the vital principle is the same for all living beings, and is shaped like two entwined serpents (or a vine, a rope or a ladder). This ability is the source of their astonishing botanical and medicinal knowledge. The way they access this knowledge is through what Narby calls defocalized and 'non rational' states of consciousness, otherwise known as ASCs. The results are empirically verifiable. The myths of many of the cultures he studied, and I have researched, are filled with biological imagery. He also compared the shamanic metaphorical explanations to the descriptions biologists are starting to provide, and found that they correspond quite precisely.

The Hawaiian Mystical System

Huna, or more appropriately, Ho'omana, is an ancient Hawaiian system of healing and preventative medicine (*Wesselman, 2011*). It provides a vehicle to help understand how the human mind, body, and spirit all work together to maintain wellness and health.

Shamanic training in Polynesia was either formal or informal, depending on the area. In New Zealand, Maori candidates attended a psychic school or Whare Wanagnga, where they underwent rigorously controlled training and examinations.

The Hawaiian system was much more family orientated, with candidates being selected from the family or even adopted into the family of a master shaman, where they were trained informally by the shaman. In the Maori tradition, students were given specific things to accomplish and were tested on them. In the Hawaiian system, they were given experiences, demonstrations and hints, and then left to develop their own experiences and discipline. This is akin to some of the Native American shamanic traditions, and places significantly more onus on the student.

The Hawaiian shaman is deemed to be a 'releaser of blocks', and was trained in the release of energy to relieve physical, emotional and mental stress, and in methods of changing limiting beliefs. Energy release was most often based on lomi-lomi, a form of massage that combines many elements of acupressure, Swedish, and Esalen massage, Rolfing, and polarity therapy. However, personal and environmental geomancy was also used for such release. The dissolving of limiting beliefs is done in a number of ways, but the most common method used was a kind of talk therapy often including affirmations. The shamans were also manifesters, shapeshifters, peacemakers, and teachers.

At the end of the nineteenth century, Dr William Tufts Brigham first began to uncover these long lost methods. He called this body of knowledge Huna. This is the name now used by most Westerners who have come to know elements of the system of Hawaiian Mysticism. Brigham initiated Max Freedom Long into the system around 1920 (*Freedom Long,1955*). This soon became Freedom Long's lifetime work until he died in 1972. He published many works on 'Huna' and began a network of Huna Research Associates around the world. He wrote extensively, and it is largely through his efforts that elements of the ancient Hawaiian Mysticism are very much alive today in the Western world, (*Huna Bulletins, 2008*). His work has its place in the development of the Western understanding of Hawaiian

Mysticism, however it is important to acknowledge that this is somewhat removed from the indigenous teachings of the ancient Hawaiian tradition.

This is brought to light in the relationship between Hank Wesselman and a Hawaiian elder with whom he was working and developing a deep friendship. (*Wesselman, 2011*). Early in their relationship, Hank, in his enthusiasm, shared the name of his friend in a newsletter. The elder, an authentically initiated kahuna had no wish to see his name in print. However, once Hank apologised for his western zeal, the relationship was put back on track, and ultimately permission was given to write a book about their friendship (*The Bowl of Light, 2011*).

During his time in Hawaii in the late nineteenth and early twentieth centuries, Dr Brigham was the curator of the Bishop Museum in Honolulu. He met many kahunas, (the word means 'Keeper of the Secret') who, although outlawed by the government, worked among their fellow Hawaiians as healers. These were remarkable people, some of whom fire-walked over lava flows which were barely cooled enough to take their weight, and others, demonstrated instant healing. After observing such 'miracles', Dr Brigham concluded that there must be a single basic scientific system lying behind these phenomena. The kahunas had a strict cult of secrecy and were reluctant to share their knowledge. However, Brigham slowly began to piece together the clues he found, and to compile a body of knowledge (*Huna Bulletins, 2008*) that lead him to the following conclusions:

- There must be a form, entity, or monad of consciousness which was in man or without him, and which the kahunas were able to contact through ceremony or prayer.
- This unidentified consciousness could use an unidentified force in such a way as to control temperature in fire-walking or make changes in physical matter creating instant healing.

After Brigham died, Max Freedom Long continued the research and work. Finally, in 1935, new clues emerged which led to him identifying what he believed to be the basic system of instantaneous healing. These new 'clues' came fundamentally from the study of the meaning of the roots of Hawaiian words. Other research, most notably that of Dr Alexis Carrel (1935), also supported the concept of instant healing in other parts of the world. The most numerous occurrences of such healings have been verified, and studied in Lourdes, France. Each appears to be accompanied by a specific prayer.

In Hawaii, the kahunas would roughly set a bone and chant a prayer, and apparently, the patient could immediately use the injured limb. One such documented method was described by J.A.K. Combs of Honolulu (*Huna Bulletins, 2008*); his wife's kahuna grandmother healed a compound fracture of the ankle using this method. Max Freedom Long concluded that no particular 'god' had to be prayed to, and no particular religious beliefs were needed. He further concluded that three things were necessary for instant healing and/or fire-walking.

1. An intelligence wise enough to bring about healing or temperature changes when requested to do so.
2. Some force or power which is used in making the changes.
3. The substances; which are changed in the healing process.

In addition there are substances which are involved in the making and offering of the prayer. These form a basic triad; Mind-Force-Matter. In the Huna system, there are nine elements in man. Mind is a triad of grades of consciousness; Force is a triad of voltages of force; Matter is a triad of densities of a kind of thin matter.

Slowly, the kahunas revealed more of their knowledge to Max Freedom Long. Although we now know that a great deal of information and knowledge was not shared. The diagram below sets out the three selves according to the Huna tradition.

According to Freedom Long (1983), the kahunas considered man to be composed of three 'selves', the Aumakua which is

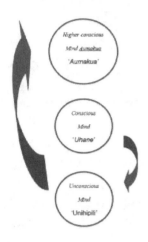

described as our Christ Consciousness, the Uhane that is our conscious self and the Unihipili, our unconscious or subconscious self. The only way to access our Aumakua is through our Unihipili (as shown above). All illness was seen by the kahunas as a disconnection between the three selves, and as the Aumakua holds the blueprint of perfect health, if we lose this connection, we create dis-ease.

He also states that the Aumakua constructs the future; it lays out the main points of the life of the individual of which it is part. Furthermore, the day-to-day future is created by taking the thoughts, hopes, fears and plans

Fig 5: Levels of the Self (Silverthorn, and Overdurf, 1999)

of the Unihipili and Uhane. These two selves plant the 'seeds' from which we grow the events of our tomorrows. We have free will in that we think what we choose, get into trouble, and do as we please, creating our future and life events. We therefore exercise free will except for the determination of the long-term events of our lives, such as birth, race, and place.

According to Hale Kealohalani Makua, Hank Wesselman's friend and mentor in Hawaiian Mysticism (The Bowl of Light, 2011), our Aumakua is our immortal soul. He said that our Aumakua is a vibration, and that each part of the word has a meaning. 'Makua' means parent, and 'au' means time, so our personal 'Aumakua', your Higher Self, is your parent, your ancestor in time.

The kahunas said that instant healing is created by deciding that we want a future that is healed (*Steiger, 1973*). (This is a similar concept to that of shapeshifting the future as discussed in the section on Shapeshifting.) If we ask the Aumakua to heal a broken bone instantly, and it is done, the kahunas say that the Aumakua has changed the future. The point to be made here is that we are free agents and must decide what we want, and to hold that decision, as an initial step in obtaining help from the Aumakua.

The Aumakua, according to Max Freedom Long, in one of his bulletins (*Huna Bulletins, 2008*) is not hampered by reason or memory as it functions on a higher plane than the forms of mentation we use at the conscious (Uhane) and unconscious (Unihipili) levels. This form of mentation used by Aumakua cannot be understood at lower levels of consciousness.

Freedom Long says that all we can do is to observe the things that Aumakua is able to do, and then to draw whatever conclusions we are able. He says that God is unknowable to us and that Aumakua can be known in part. He uses the analogy of the relationship between a man and his dog. The man cares for the dog and plans the 'must' dos such as feeding and exercise. The dog can then do what she pleases most of the time. She may get into trouble and run to her master for help. The master understands his dog, and the dog knows a lot about her master, but because she has a dog's mind, many of the activities and purposes of her master must remain mysteries. This is very like the relationship between Uhane and Aumakua.

In Hawaiian Mysticism, all things are triune. There is always,

- A consciousness being used
- A force or power, to work with
- Some form of matter, either dense or etheric matter

The Aumakua lives external to, and yet connected with the physical body, whereas Uhane and Unihipili reside within the physical body. Hawaiian Mysticism recognizes three levels or voltages of vital force, one level for each of the three selves (*Lawrence & Lawrence 1994*). These energies are known as mana, mana-mana, and Mana-Loa. The teachings show that these energies of healing are the same energies as our life force. They are a part of our being, and surround us as long as we are living. They can be transformed and regenerated but can never be destroyed.

Kahunas called the primary energy, mana; this is the energy of Unihipili. It is our life force, and is created by the interaction of the food we eat and the oxygen we breathe. Mana is low vibration energy; it is essential for the maintenance and daily operation of our body. Without mana we would become cold and die, for it is mana that runs our biological systems. It provides us with the energy to live life, and ultimately heal ourselves. It is also the energy of the stress mechanism.

Mana-mana is the energy of Uhane and our willpower. In the Hawaiian language when a word is doubled, it signifies that it is greater than its original form. Hence, mana-mana is of greater energy and has a higher vibrational energy than mana. The mana-mana of Uhane is stronger than mana alone and yet it still cannot connect to the Aumakua. Mana-mana is also generated by food and breathing, and it powers our desires and intentional activities. Without willpower we would have no mechanism for getting what we want in life.

Mana-mana is the power of our consciousness and allows us to have free will. Mana has its own biological functions, and it is also affected directly by the commands of Uhane. Mana-mana can either be broad or narrow sighted. As will or desire it can be mixed with emotions, and react to internal feelings and emotions long forgotten by conscious memory. It can act on Unihipili as a benevolent friend or as a demi-god force, out of its own belief and in its own cause.

Mana-Loa is the energy of Aumakua, and it is often thought of as a psychic energy or spiritual energy. According to Lawrence and Lawrence (*1994*), it resonates at a vibrational level higher than either mana, or mana-mana. Mana-Loa acts differently than either of the other two energies. It is directly involved in prayer, including healing and desiring prayers as well as providing our connection to the intelligence of the universe. Through the process of prayer, mana-mana, as willpower, decision, or commitment, is sent to Unihipili. If Unihipili accepts the prayer, and is not blocked by fear, guilt, or other complexes, then mana is activated and sent through an Aka cord (energy connection) from Unihipili to Aumakua. When Aumakua accepts the prayer, mana-loa is activated and creates what was asked for in the prayer.

Occasionally, Unihipili will recognize a higher truth, and lets this truth into its level of consciousness. In these instances, it may become immediately energized by its own passion of being. A doorway then opens, and a spontaneous enlightenment may occur. When this happens, mana is involuntarily sent up to Aumakua, Mana-Loa is produced and healing takes place. The person enters into an altered state of consciousness (ASC), which allows the healing to occur. I have had several personal experiences of this whilst I was learning various shamanic practices, and have worked with numerous clients using a range of shamanic techniques where such instantaneous healings have occurred.

These three energies can be abused and often are. When this occurs the person affected will often say that they have 'no energy', and they feel tired or depressed. What is actually happening is that energy is being drawn from the lower (Unihipili) and middle (Uhane) selves. In other words, their energies have been misdirected or drawn off into unhelpful tasks such as worrying, and the suppression of emotions such as guilt, fears or anxieties. When someone is feeling limited in some way they tend to allocate their energy poorly. For example, energy, which would normally be used to activate the immune system, may be misdirected into worrying about a problem that they are fearful of solving. The result will often be minor ailments, which can become compounded if this continues, and may result in more serious disease. As western medicine in general does not recognize, or have an understanding of the role of life force energy, people with energy problems are often diagnosed as suffering from chronic fatigue, immune system deficiency or depression.

Breath and Healing

In Hawaiian Mysticism, as with a number of other philosophies, breathing is fundamental. If we don't breathe we die; however, many of us have forgotten how to breathe properly. I recall a time when I was visiting Hawaii with my former husband. I had recently passed my diving exams and we planned to do some diving. I had quite a traumatic time during my diver training, and had experienced great difficulty in breathing due to the tightness of my wet suit. So, I was a little anxious about getting back into the water.

We were walking along the street one afternoon when a Hawaiian man came up to me and said very loudly, 'Breathe.' I nearly jumped out of my skin, which is probably what I needed to do! Then the following day we went to a performance of Ula'hena (a beautiful depiction of Hawaiian legend in dance). As we stood in the lobby, one of the actors came up and said, 'Breathe, lady, breathe. I got the message; my anxiety was causing me to breathe very shallowly and was literally weakening my energy. Sadly, this is common place in our society as many people only use the very top part of their lungs to breathe and do not receive the energetic benefits of full, deep breathing, which brings balance to our lives.

According to Lawrence and Lawrence (1994), breathing provides the following benefits:

- It cleanses the system, removes toxins from the blood stream
- Brings in oxygen, generating energy to burn food
- Reduces stress
- Works the muscles of the diaphragm and abdomen
- Increases blood flow to the heart
- Increases oxygen circulation throughout the body
- Increases oxygen to the brain
- Improves blood sugar usage

In my own experience, clients who are stressed and anxious are breathing very shallowly, and sometimes their breathing is barely visible it is so shallow. The first thing I do is get them to stop and take a few long, slow, deep breaths. This causes them to alter their state of consciousness, so that we can begin our work together. At present in mainstream western medicine, physicians are not taught how to connect breathing with healing. So the connection of breath to the generation of body energy (mana and mana-mana) and spiritual healing energy, Mana-Loa, is not made.

A kahuna uses 'supercharged' energy to directly heal, to return the physical system to balance, and to overcome problems of blocked energy. This is achieved through the use of specific prayers. He or she also knows that proper breathing, and the ability to direct the breathing process is imperative to the production of energy.

Breathing is important not only for our biological processes but also because of its other effects on the mind, body, and spirit. Students of Hawaiian Mysticism realize this early in their training and use breath to evaluate an individual. The way someone breathes, the depth of their breath, and their breathing patterns are all key indicators of their well-being. In the example I gave of myself above, I was clearly not in a state of well-being. In western medicine these indicators are generally ignored except in extreme situations such as shock, or in chronic conditions such as asthma.

Aka

In Hawaiian Mysticism the three energies of the body also have physical counterparts; often these are referred to as auras, astral bodies, or etheric bodies, these are called the aka bodies. Each of the bodies are separate, and yet interconnected. For instance, when mana is sent to the Aumakua it moves through an aka cord. This is a cord of aka material that connects the aka body of the Unihipili to the aka body of the Aumakua. There is also an aka cord that connects the aka body of the Uhane and the Unihipili. (See diagram above.)

In mythology the aka cord is also known as the silver cord. This attaches our aka body to our physical body. The concept of astral travel relies on the ability of the aka bodies of the Uhane and Unihipili to leave the physical body, and to travel wherever they desire. As long as the silver cord remains intact, the aka bodies of the Uhane and Unihipili can return to the physical body at any time. If, however, it is cut or breaks for any reason, the aka bodies are unable to return to the physical body. It is the silver cord that is severed during the process of dying, preventing the aka bodies from returning to the physical. The result is the irrevocable loss of life force. This function is also in process when people have a Near Death Experience (NDE). Many doctors refuse to believe that someone can die and return to life having experienced 'the other side'. For those of us who are students of shamanism, we have been taught that as the life force begins to ebb, the aka bodies of the Unihipili and Uhane separate out and leave the physical body, but the silver cord remains intact.

In 2002, I had been a student of Hawaiian Mysticism for several years when I had a Near Death Experience (NDE). I had learned about the aka bodies and silver cord. When I had my NDE, I recall being totally fascinated by seeing my apparently lifeless body lying face down in a ditch with a silver cord attaching my physical body to the 'me' floating above it.

According to one of my teachers, Kahuna Uncle George Naope, the aka bodies are exact duplicates of the physical. The aka body of the Unihipili has memories but lacks the ability or the logic to make decisions. The aka body of the Uhane has no memories but can make decisions, and when away from the physical body and in a solid form, could easily be mistaken for the individual him or herself.

According to physician Dr Allen Lawrence (1994), the beliefs of the physician have an impact on the health of his or her patients. He says that when we believe in something we give it power. So, if a doctor does not believe his patient will get well, the likelihood is that they will not recover unless the patient's beliefs to the contrary are stronger than that of the doctor. Unfortunately, this is rare, as the majority of people see a doctor as an authority in health and disease. In hypnosis, we say that this places the doctor in a position of prestige, and creates something that is called 'prestige suggestibility'. The patient is hence in a position where they are open to suggestion simply because they view the doctor as the authority. Since most illness and disease are simply an intelligent message from the body (Unihipili) communicating conflict, then indeed, these illnesses are, according to Dr Lawrence, illusions. This is why he says that enlightened physicians can never believe in illness nor give up on a patient until death has occurred. If he or she recognizes illness as an illusion, he or she is aware that below the illusion there is a truth that must be found to create wellness.

In this philosophy, when we become ill we are creating an illusion. If our Uhane believes in the illusion sufficiently it can completely miss the message from our Unihipili that we have an internal conflict. If we persistently ignore this message, our Unihipili will also eventually believe in the illness. And if Uhane continually tells Unihipili that the illness is real, then both will eventually tell our Aumakua, and our Aumakua will manifest the illness we have 'asked for'. This happens without finding the cause and solving the necessary problems; therefore, the process of illness progresses. Eventually this robs us of our health and vitality, and if not stopped, could ultimately kill us.

Once Unihipili is convinced by Uhane that illness exists, it begins to 'act out' the illness or disease (dis-ease). Initially, this triggers the stress mechanism and when it finds no tangible illness, it begins to turn against itself, creating allergies, autoimmune disease, and so on. Eventually, it may break down in a kind of metabolic exhaustion. With the immune system impaired, the body's defence mechanisms are 'instructed' that they must allow this to happen (Unihipili believes that what is happening is real), this sets the stage for the person to become truly ill, and once in the body, the illness takes on a life of its own. Dr Lawrence goes on to say, that if the ill person goes to see a doctor, he may go to a doctor who believes in the illness. If this occurs, the doctor's beliefs combined with his own belief in the illness can create a situation where the progression of the illness is accepted. If, however, he goes to a doctor who does not believe in the illness or who believes strongly in the possibility of a cure, and the patient accepts the doctor's ability to cure him, he may rapidly get better.

Kahunas use a form of prayer to create healing. By uncovering the hidden reasons for the illness, defining the problem and finding ways to solve it, the process of the illness can be reversed and health can be restored. This only makes sense when the illness is thought of as an intelligent act of the body as it attempts to communicate conflict that is not being resolved (*Lawrence & Lawrence 1994*). The illness is seen here as an act of wisdom of the body/mind in working to resolve a conflict.

The first step in the Hawaiian process of healing is to change our beliefs about something. However, it is fundamentally important that we create a specific healing prayer created by Uhane (our conscious self). This confirms our decision to get well and passes the message on to Unihipili. Usually, Unihipili sees this prayer as a new command from Uhane, and will change the bodily processes such as the immune system's ability to respond or function. The prayer also acts on Unihipili so that it combines the prayer statement (a seed) with a vital force (mana), and sends these two together up to Aumakua. This process establishes a pathway for creating positive images for the future, and will lead to a cure with the resolution of the signs and symptoms associated with the original conflict.

In Hawaiian a traditional prayer is seen as planting a seed; a thought form of wellness. This is akin to the fact that when we plant an acorn we expect an oak tree to grow. The acorn (the seed) contains the nature of what is to grow from it. Prayer works in the same way, a thought form that is carefully constructed will generate what is expected from it. Our thoughts are considered to be packets of energy with form, shape, and substance. The same is said to be true about our ideas and beliefs as they are also thought forms. It is essential that we are very clear about what we ask for, because we will create this in our lives. Therefore, we create a very specific picture of whatever we desire, and ask for it in the faith that we are getting it. The picture includes all the submodalities of feelings and sounds, as well as visual images. (This has been adapted and used in the NLP technique of Time Line Therapy™.)

The Hawaiian Mystical symbol of the thought form is the seed. For the seed to grow into a mature plant, giving us what we want, we must nurture and water it. To ensure this, it is important that we do everything necessary to make our thought form blossom into what is expected from it. This applies to all thoughts, ideas and beliefs, as each one is a seed. Each can grow and reach fruition. It is important that every day we send a daily charge of mana to Aumakua to enable the seeds we have planted to grow. The symbol for mana is water, which when given to the seeds (thought forms) will enable them to grow. Our faith in the final outcome is like the soil, substance, or earth in which we plant the seed. Ultimately the key to having the life that we want lies in our thoughts, ideas, and beliefs, and of equal importance, the words we use to ask for them. Once again the linguistics learned in NLP is a vital tool in enabling us to ask for the things we want in a very clear and precise way, ensuring that there is no room for misinterpretation.

Prayer

A prayer acts as a petition from Uhane directly to Unihipili, and if necessary on to the Aumakua. The clearest understanding of a Hawaiian prayer is provided for us in the New Testament, where Jesus tells us, 'Ask and you shall receive, seek and you shall find.' The difference between what we are taught about prayer in our western culture and the Hawaiian prayer is that when making a prayer we understand what we are doing, we plan and prepare the prayer to ask for whatever we desire. The underlying principle here is that we will receive whatever we desire, and create in this way as long as it causes no hurt or harm to ourselves, or others.

In creating our specific prayer we must first decide what we want, and write out our prayer. It is paramount that we write the prayer clearly, in language that creates the image of that which we want to create (without the use of negative language). We must then find a calm peaceful place to present the prayer, so that both Unihipili and Uhane can focus on the prayer. A good example of this is taken from one of Max Freedom Long's Letters on Huna (*1949-1971*):

I ask for the strength to open my eyes and my heart to see what I previously feared to see. As I see my conflicts, I will set them straight. I will take full responsibility for the problems

I caused. I return my life to full and complete wellness and health. These blurred and confused conditions have been the cause of my vision problems. I now give praise to my eyes, my mind, and my body for giving me evidence of these conflicts. From this moment on I see perfectly. As I saw my conflicts, I presently see in absolute clarity all that is around me, today, tomorrow and everyday in the future. I see perfectly and normally in every way, and I shall continue to see perfectly well all of my life.

Tradition suggests that a prayer of the Hawaiian Mystical tradition is repeated at least three times, calmly and clearly. This repetition is important as it reinforces to the lower self (Unihipili) that this is something important. It is also important that the prayer be said congruently, so that Unihipili believes what we say and sends the message up to Aumakua. We also need to have faith and to believe that this will be, believing that it will occur when it is ready to manifest.

To ensure that our prayers work properly and quickly, several steps are required (*Lawrence & Lawrence 1994*):

1. The use of the prayer must be accepted, believed, and truly desired.
2. The prayer-action must be practised until our Unihipili has learned the work that it must do.
3. Repetition is extremely valuable. The prayers work best if repeated at least three times a day.
4. Before starting the prayer, amends must be made for all hurts done to others. This enables feelings of negativity to drop away.
5. What is asked for must be for the good of all concerned and must hurt no one.
6. It is always helpful to pray for others or for healing of others, however, when prayer is confused or cluttered it

is less likely to come to fruition.

7. The more love, self respect and self-esteem we feel and experience for our self and others, the more likely the prayer will be fulfilled.

A prayer action is ended when it feels as though the message has been passed to, and been accepted by Aumakua. Often, this acceptance is associated with a profound sense of joy (ASC). I was also taught to use my breath to send the mana to Aumakua. Therefore, I take three deep breaths, inhaling and exhaling slowly and deeply at the end of each prayer. It feels as if I am literally breathing life into the prayer. For people who are new to this, it may not be easily discernable, so the best advice is to repeat it three times. It is important to let the prayer settle, so remaining relaxed for about an hour afterwards, allows Unihipili to carry out our instructions rather than running immediately on to the next tasks for the day.

Ho'oponopono.

According to the teachings of Morrnah K Simeona, originally taught to my former husband Robert Moeller in 1989, there are twelve steps to the Ho'oponopono process (*Simeona, 1980*). Morrnah was a renowned Kahuna who is credited with bringing the modern form of Ho'oponopono to her students.

The twelve steps she developed were:

1. The inner connection – the focus for this step is connecting Uhane with the Aumakua. It is principally a prayer from Uhane to Aumakua through Unihipili. The prayer asks Unihipili, the child, to forgive the actions of Uhane, thoughts, words, and deeds. It asks Unihipili to hold hands with (join with) Uhane to connect with Aumakua. It asks for love to flow from Uhane, to Unihipili and to Aumakua, embracing all three in a divine circle of love.

2. 'For I am Peace' – the focus for this step is 'I'. This is a process to gently release fear. It is a slow and gentle process to reach Unihipili. We are invited by Aumakua to enter into silent solitude, and let go of all emotions. Once we have done this we feel a letting go, and affirm that we are a child of God, allowing Divine Love and Intelligence to flow through us. We acknowledge that we are always in the right place at the right time for our growth, personal success, and happiness, allowing us to use our talents for our own good and the good of others. It ends with the statement, 'I am Peace'.

3. Breathing (HA) –
   - Inhale (Divine Energy) for the count of 7
   - Hold breath for the count of 7
   - Exhale for the count of 7
   - Hold breath for the count of 7
   (This is repeated 9 times)

4. Opening prayer, I am the 'I' supplement – the following prayer is said,
   'I' come forth from the void into the light,
   'I' am the breath that nurtures life,
   'I' am that emptiness, that hollowness beyond all consciousness
   The 'I', the id, the all,
   'I' draw my bow of rainbows across the waters,
   The continuum of mind with matters,
   'I' am the incoming and outgoing of breath,
   The invisible, untouchable breeze,
   The undefinable atom of creation,
   'I' am the 'I'.

5. Repentance prayer – this is a prayer between the individual (or a group) and the Divine Creator. The prayer asks for forgiveness for all the wrongs we, our family, and ancestors have committed. It ends with,

'AND IT IS DONE'. This signals that this is where Man's work ends and God's work begins.

6. Ho'oponopono; the long form, or short form; conception and Mahiki.

The long form is in two parts. The first part is a prayer that asks for forgiveness for all our wrong doings and asks that the Divine Intelligence include anything we may have omitted. The second part asks that Divine Order, light, love, balance, wisdom, understanding, and abundance be made manifest in our lives.

The short form compresses this all into one step.

The conception prayer is included to heal any trauma associated with any abortions or miscarriages, releasing them into the light.
The Mahiki prayer is for the cleansing and releasing of negative vibrations from people, entities, atoms, and molecules. They are released into pure light.

7. Release – this prayer cuts all our aka cords (all our connections) with all things, people, and places, releasing us, and setting us free.

8. Cleanse – this prayer mentally bathes us in indigo, emerald green, ice blue, and white light. We envisage these lights each bathing our body 7 times.

9. Transmute – this prayer asks the Divine Intelligence to release and transmute all toxins, and negative vibrations into pure light.

10. Closing prayer – The Peace of 'I',
    Peace be with you, all my peace
    The Peace that is 'I', the peace that is 'I am',
    The peace for always and now and forever and ever more,

> My peace 'I' give to you, My peace 'I' leave with you,
> Not the world's peace, but only my peace, the peace of
> 'I'.

11. Breathing (HA) – 7 rounds (as bullet 3 above).
12. Acknowledgements – this is a prayer acknowledging all the Aumkuas, Unihipilis and Uhanes involved in the Ho'oponopono process, the divine forces of all living things, the Aumakuas of the world, universe, and cosmos.

I have used this form of Ho'oponopono on numerous occasions, especially when moving house or when there is a potentially challenging time ahead. Each time I experience a significant shift in my consciousness and feel a sense of peace and tranquillity. The events have panned out smoothly in each instance.

Tad James also taught me a more simplified Ho'oponopono process at my NLP Master Practitioner training in 1996. In this version, I was taught to create a stage in my imagination and to bring all the people in my life onto this stage one by one. The process involves telling each person how we feel about them, then to send them love, sever the aka cords connecting us, and send the person off into the Light. It was recommended that we do this each night before going to sleep as it breaks the existing energetic connection that we have with those people. This leaves us free to reconnect with those people in the way we would like to connect with them, (if indeed we want to reconnect) rather than in the old energetic way in which we were previously connected. I have also found this to be a powerful process, which I continue to use on a regular basis. It is amazing how many times I have done this only to find that the person in question will often call or email me within 24 hours.

Fire Walking

I had the privilege of being trained as a fire walk instructor in 2002 by Peggy Dylan. Peggy along with her ex husband, Tolly

Burkan, is renowned for the introduction of fire walking to the Western World in the 1970s. I found this to be a personally very healing, and transformative process. There are a number of theories about how it is possible to walk on red-hot coals or lava without being burned; however, there is yet to be validated scientific evidence to fully explain how we can do this.

The most common theory is that when we raise our energy to match the energy of the fire, we are able to walk safely across the coals with no physical damage to our feet. Some people have stated that the only way this can be done is through hypnosis. The other side of this argument is that while it could be possible for hypnotized people to walk across the coals without feeling pain, hypnosis in of itself would not prevent the skin from being burned. As mentioned in the section on Huna, Dr Brigham experienced walking across a barely cooled lava flow with two kahunas. He had refused to take off his boots, when he got to the other side the soles of his heavy walking boots had been burned off, yet there was no damage to his feet.

The eminent doctor and healer, Andrew Weil, describes his experience of fire walking,

> ...you can walk in some other state of mind-body in which sensation and tissue responses are different from normal. Encouraging you to find that 'altered state' where your mind, and even your body, are under your control, is what this book is all about. Knowing that I hadn't attained it with my first walk, I wanted to try again. (*Burkan,* 2004)

According to Wikipedia, the on line encyclopedia, (*www. wikipedia.com*) the oldest recorded fire walk occurred over 4,000 years ago in India. Apparently, two Brahmin priests had a competition to see who could walk the longest distance over hot coals. The victor's triumph was written down and this record apparently still exists today. In the 17th century, a Jesuit priest,

Father Le Jeune, wrote a report to his superior, describing a healing fire walk he witnessed among the North American Indians. He reported that a sick woman walked through two or three hundred fires with bare legs and feet. She did not burn, and said that she could feel no uncomfortable heat. Similarly another priest, Father Marquette reported seeing similar fire walks among the Ottawa Indians.

Furthermore, Jonathon Carver writes in his 1802 book, *Travels in North America* that one of the most astounding sights he saw was the parade of warriors who would 'walk naked through a fire... with apparent immunity'.

Variable forms of fire worship as a rite of healing, purification, initiation, and transcendence have woven a thread through our cultural tapestry for millennia.

Today, many indigenous peoples have, or indeed had, various rituals and ceremonies in honour of fire, its sacred powers, and gifts. Through the centuries, fire worship, and fire walking as key aspects of the sacredness of fire have continued to play their role in nurturing the human spirit. In our twenty-first century western world, fire walking is often used as a powerful tool for personal transformation, especially as a healing process.

If we look to nature, we see the cleansing and purifying aspects of wild fires, when they clear the way for the new growth that many animal and plant species depend upon for life. Some seeds require the heat of fire to enable them to break through their shells and grow, and in much the same way, human beings can benefit from the power of fire. Fire produces nutrients more quickly than decay, many pine cones require the heat of a fire to pop open and free their seeds; grasslands burn to get rid of the stubble which shades and crowds new life, and birds like the endangered red-cockaded woodpecker thrive only in areas regularly burned.

According to Peggy Dylan, (2002) our relationship with fire is as old as the human race. She states that recent evidence suggests that Australopithecus controlled fire nearly a million and a half years ago. While the absolute beginnings of fire walking are unknown, the earliest documentation found originates from the seventeenth century. What is known is that Africa, often considered the birthplace of mankind, has a long history of both fire walking and fire dancing.

The !Kung Bushmen of the Kalahari desert have long incorporated fire walking as an inherent part of their culture, which can actually be traced back to their cultural origins. They use a fire walk as an integral part of their powerful healing ceremonies. Likewise, African born Hindus have a history of walking on fire as a part of their important religious festivals.

In 1977, Laurens Van Der Post, (*New Edition 2002*) the renowned anthropologist published an account of his travels into the Kalahari Desert, and his studies of the !Kung. He says he was amazed when he first witnessed their healing fire dances. In addition, Richard Katz, a psychologist at Harvard reports (1984) that the !Kung use fire to heat up their energy, which they call n/um. The dancers go to the fire where they walk on it, put their heads in it, and pick up coals which they rub over their hands and body. They say that when the n/um in the body is boiling, no matter how hot the fire is, they will not be burned. He also says that as the n/um intensifies, the fire walkers experience an enhanced consciousness (ASC) which they call '!kia'. At this point, they know they are able to heal all those at the fire walk, whether they are walking or not.

According to one North American Indian legend, (Dylan, 2002) fire was first sparked by buffalo hooves thundering across the plains. The Maoris of New Zealand believe it was a gift from a god's blind grandmother, who drew it from her fingernails by magic. In the legends of the Huachipayri Indians of the Amazon basin in Peru, a woodpecker brought fire. They still call his name and imitate his call when making fire with fire sticks in their ceremonies.

In Bali, it is the young girls who dance on the fire. In India, Sri Lanka, Tibet, China, Japan, North America, and Argentina for instance, people walk and dance joyously, exuberantly, or devotionally across the fire. In Agni Hotra, the Hindu fire ceremony, fire is used to purify the physical and spiritual energy. Similarly in Peru, the flame is used for spiritual uplifting in their fire ceremonies. In North America, several shamanic cultures such as the Fox, Menomini, Kere, Blackfoot, and Zuni are known to have a 'great fire fraternity'. Moreover, as mentioned in the section on Huna, some kahunas had a healing practice which included walking across lava. As with many shamanic practices there are variations of fire walking throughout the world, each practice is designed to bring the participants closer to their true nature, enabling them to heal and be renewed.

In the late 1970s and early 1980s, Tolly Burkan and Peggy Dylan began their work of re-introducing fire walking into the western world. Since that time fire walking has become an acceptable tool for corporate seminars, and has created something of a cult following in the rapidly expanding personal growth and development industry. From my own perspective, this increased awareness of fire walking has come at some cost, as many of the trainings have lost sight of the spiritual and shamanic roots of the practice. People enter a high energy state (ASC) to walk the fire, but lose the vast healing benefits, which if they do occur, are a side benefit because the main focus is one of 'conquering' the fire.

Interestingly, the incidence of reported burns in newspapers and on the Internet, have increased quite dramatically with the increasing popularity of sponsored evening fire walks. Most of these events consist of a brief talk followed by the fire walk. This type of brief event does not allow sufficient time for effective preparation to enable people to receive the full personal and group healing benefits of a fire walk. The intention is usually to get people to walk across the hot coals to raise money for charity, which in itself is laudable, however it is in danger of reducing the fire walk to something significantly less than its true potential as a transformational tool. Hence, this also increases the risk of people being burned.

As a fire walk instructor I know that a person's attitude as they approach the fire will affect whether they are able to walk, and if they do walk, if they will hurt themselves or not. When including fire walking in my training workshops, I am acutely aware of the importance of preparing people for their walk, and to create an atmosphere of healing. I am very careful to explain that rather than conquering the fire, the purpose is to build an energetic partnership with the fire, to allow our n/um to merge with that of the fire, so that we can walk safely, and hence allow the energy of the fire to heal us. Those people who feel that they need to conquer the fire are missing the point. This is an adversarial approach, and one, which often results in people burning themselves. This is because they oppose the energy of the fire rather than working with it.

It is also important that people decide for themselves when, and if, they walk on the coals. In my own experience, and from feedback from course participants, there comes a point when we know we are ready to walk. The first time I ever did a fire walk was with a very famous seminar leader at a weekend programme in London. There were over 8,000 people there and 35 lines of fire. It was like being at a cattle market rather than a healing and spiritually uplifting experience. There is no doubt that the energy was high, palpably so, but it was personally a non-event. There was someone at the beginning of the fire who told those of us in line when we were ready to walk. The woman in front of me was sent to the back of the line as she was deemed 'unready'. I was then told to go across the coals. I reached the other side with a feeling of uncertainty and confusion; my feet were then sprayed with cold water from a hose pipe. To me this represented great organisation but a complete absence of the purpose of doing something as potentially transformational as a fire walk. I was left with a feeling of emptiness. This sent me on a mission to find an authentic fire walking experience.

When I undertook my apprenticeship with Peggy Dylan, I discovered that the energy builds inside of us as our consciousness shifts, and there is an 'internal knowing' when it is the right time to walk. People who at the outset have said that they would not walk but would like to join the healing energy, song, and dance around the fire, report all of a sudden knowing that they 'had to walk the coals'. When people reach the far side of the fire for the first time, they release huge amounts of energy, usually in the form of whoops of joy or tears. It is as if the release created by the raising of their n/um enables them to let go of any energetic blocks to healing. While this is currently an observation rather than a scientific 'truth', something definitely happens. Many people report healings from such diverse dis-eases as ME, asthma, psoriasis, high blood pressure and many more after they have walked on red hot coals as a part of a healing ceremony.

Stephen Pyne, an Arizona State University historian, who has studied fire all of his life is quoted in *National Geographic, September 1996*, as saying: 'We are uniquely fire creatures on a uniquely fire planet. Our planet is primed for ignition, "stuffed with organic fuels, its atmosphere saturated with oxygen, its surface pummeled by lightning". Many of the natural environments of our planet are dependent on the cleansing and purifying aspects of fire.'

The Anastenarian Approach

Loring Dansford's research *(1989)* into fire walking provides us with an interpretation of the Anastenaria, a northern Greek ritual involving fire walking and spirit possession, which is performed by a group of refugees from eastern Thrace. These people are known as the Kostilides, who settled in Greek Macedonia in the early 1920s. The ritual cycle of the Anastenaria in the village of

Ayia Eleni, where the largest group of Kostilides settled, reaches its climax on May 21st, the day the Orthodox Church celebrates the festival of Saints Constantine and Helen. The Anastenarides believe that Saint Constantine has the power to cause and heal a variety of illnesses. They also believe that it is Saint Constantine who possesses them when they dance, and protects them from being burned when they perform their impressive acts of fire walking.

Dansford reports that at these religious ceremonies people meet, and talk, and it is where they pay homage to the saints. It is also where some people become 'possessed', and healings take place. People travel long distances to participate in the ceremonies, or simply to watch the other people participating in what has become the spectacle of Anastenaria.

The Anastenaria is deemed to be a form of healing in the broadest sense. It combines religious ritual with a form of psychotherapy. Hence, any interpretation to understand the Anastenaria as a system of religious healing needs to combine approaches from medical anthropology with those of the anthropological study of religion. It brings together the connections between transcultural psychiatry and symbolic anthropology. Dansford states, '...the task of interpretive anthropology is to make more accessible the imaginative universes in which other people live. Systems of religious healing enable people to deal with problems in a sacred manner.'

The village of Ayia Eleni, where the Anastenaria takes place is about twelve miles south of Serres in eastern Macedonia and has a population of about forty thousand. In 1976, Ayia Eleni only had a population of around seven hundred people, mainly farmers. About half of this population comprised of the refugees from Kosti in eastern Thrace. The village reaches the awareness of people throughout the area on 21st May each year when film clips of the fire walk appear on national television. As a result, several thousand people travel to Ayai Eleni to witness and participate in these celebrations. Throughout the year there are many religious festivals that lead up to, and culminate at the 21st May celebrations for Saints Constantine and Helen. A male black lamb is sacrificed for the celebration, and is not weaned from its mother until it is taken to be sacrificed at the ceremony.

In Ayai Eleni people are considered to be Anastenarides because they regularly dance and walk on the fire when 'possessed' by Saint Constantine. Another town, Langadas, situated about fifteen miles from Thessaloniki in northern Greece, also has the ritual of Anastenarides and fire walking. The Anastenarides of Langadas fire walk for three nights as a part of the May 21st celebrations for Saints Constantine and Helen. Here they sacrifice a young bull instead of a lamb.

According to Danforth (1989), it is said that in the Anastenaria religious healing is brought about by the transformation of people's personal relationship with Saint Constantine. The relationship shifts from that of illness and suffering to a positive relationship involving health and joy. The participants believe that the transformation takes place when a person becomes an Anastenaris, and hence acquires the supernatural power of the Saint.

A person's relationship with the Saint is seen as a powerful metaphor of the person's life and present situation. The importance of Saints Constantine and Helen stems back to the stories the Kostilides tell about the origins of the fire walk. One such story is that long ago the church of Saints Constantine and Helen in Kosti caught fire. As the church burned, cries were heard coming from the icons within the flames. Some people heard the cries, and ran into the burning church to rescue the icons. Neither the icons nor the people who had saved them were burned. Hence, the Anastenarides commemorate this miracle each year on May 21st by walking through fire themselves.

Another story establishes a link between the 'miraculous' vision of Constantine and the fire walk of the Anastenarides, and the town of Kosti. According to this story *(Dansforth 1989)*, Saint Constantine was a general and originally did not believe in God or religious practice. However, his mother Helen was a very religious woman. One day Constantine was fighting his enemies in Thrace near Kosti and defeated them, causing them to flee. To prevent Constantine from pursuing them they lit a vast fire, and burned down the forest, which ultimately destroyed all the old villages around Kosti. Constantine stopped in front of the fire. Then in the sky he saw a message, 'In this sign conquer!' This apparently meant that he could pass through the fires unharmed, which he did. This allegedly occurred on May 21st.

The dance of the possessed Anastenarides is seen by its followers as an expression at the somatic level of the relationship they have with Saint Constantine. This plays an important role in shaping their trance experience. The long-term goal of the therapeutic process of the Anastenaria is realized over the duration of their career as an Anastenaris, and is the transformation from illness into health. Similarly, the short-term goal realized over the course of one dance session is the transformation of a negative trance into a positive one. What initially begins as a dance expressing anxiety and tension becomes a dance that expresses the acquisition of supernatural power.

The essential feature of the ritual therapy of the Anastenarides is the creation of the 'proper relationship with Saint Constantine', and the supposed transference of his supernatural power. The dance of the possessed Anastenarides is a symbolic language that creates the tangible, bodily experience of this power. Hence, the participation of the Anastenaria is seen to empower people. It facilitates the restructuring of their problematic relationships with others, and enables them to regain control of their lives and their health.

Ken Cadigan was a fire walk leader in the USA in the 1980s *(2008)*, and has fire walked, and fire danced with the Anastenaria.

For him, however, fire walking is a spiritual experience, not necessarily a religious one. He believes that a confident, positive attitude is able to change people's brain chemistry, which in turn changes their skin chemistry, and prevents them from being burned. This is supported in part by the scientific research of people such as Dr Candace Pert *(2003)*. On his web site, Ken says,

> Fire walking is a metaphor. We need to try to understand the element of fire in our lives; we need to bring the fire home. The fire within us is a fire of transformation. We're (sic) afraid we're going to change, so we sit separately in fear and doubt. We have to try to use the fire as a mirror for the fire within ourselves. It is an open door. You can walk through fire, and you can heal your relationships.

Personal Experience

The person who tends the fire is of fundamental importance to the experience of fire walking. It is as if the person tending the fire, and the fire become one, so the person's intentions must be pure and open. As mentioned previously, on my own fire walk instructor training we received a very powerful learning.

The course participants were divided into three groups, each with a role for the evening fire walk. The first group created the initial fire, the second group raked and tended the coals, and the third group led the walk. I was a part of the final group and when we got to the fire that evening I knew something was wrong, every fibre of my being told me that it was not a fire to be walked, that somehow the fire was 'angry'. No one seemed to want to walk the fire, and after a few minutes I said that I felt we should stop and not proceed with the walk that night, as the fire was not a safe fire to walk. One or two people said that they wanted to walk, and those that did, received minor burns on their feet.

However, most people had agreed with me, and as soon as

those who wanted to walk had done so, we raked out the coals and left them to cool on their own. The learning we all received from this was that the lack of cohesion across the three groups caused the energy of the fire to be 'confused'. In some way we had allowed a sense of energetic separation to occur, and hence there was no consistency in the relationship with the fire. I would even go so far as to say that there was an element of ego and competition between the three groups to see who would 'perform' the best.

I knew at some deep level, that, no matter how much love and attention I poured into the coals that night, it was not a safe fire to walk because of all the disparate energy that had gone into creating them. It was a huge lesson for me in the effectiveness of energy transference, and the power of fire energy. As mentioned above, the people who walked that evening received some minor burns, and interestingly this is the only fire walk I have attended or led where this has occurred. Hence, that evening I received an important learning about the key role the fire keeper plays at a fire walk. They hold the energy for the group by consistently focusing their intention on creating a safe and loving fire to enable the participants to walk safely. This role is pivotal to the success of any healing and transformative fire walk.

According to Ken Cadigan (2008), fire walking brings about two different types of healing: physiological healing, here he cites examples of cancer patients going into remission after a fire walk, and psychological healing when people will complete things after a fire walk that they have been unable to finish because of fear or doubt.

In my own experience as a participant, and also as a fire walk leader, I have received a number of personal healings; one example is the eczema I had for years disappearing from my right foot. I have also witnessed people making choices to change their work, changing the location where they live, and healing conditions such as ME.

I have also learned the importance of setting clear intentions for the walk. NLP has been very powerful in assisting me and my students in setting clear objectives in language that ensures there is no doubt about the intention for people before they walk the fire. NLP enables me to coach people to ensure that the linguistics of their intentions are clean, enabling the unconscious mind to readily understand these intentions, and transmit them to our Higher Self. This enables all three selves to align and work together to achieve the desired outcome. The actual fire walk then provides the energetic vehicle for bringing the three selves together. When we know it is time to stand at the head of the fire preparing to walk, we have already entered an ASC, and suddenly it feels as if something inside knows that we are ready to walk safely. When this is done with clear intent, we are connecting through our Higher Self to the Universal consciousness; it is as if the universe conspires to help us achieve our goals.

Sun Dancing

The Sun Dance is the largest and most important ceremony in the Lakota spiritual tradition, the one that 'ensures the life of the people' for another year. One of the most well-known Sun Dance leaders is Leonard Crow Dog (referred to in the section on plant medicine), who combines many aspects of spirituality from being a minister in the Peyote Church, to leading sweat lodges and Sun Dances. For most people, this deeply sacred ceremony is only known to them through the movie staring Richard Harris in 'A Man called Horse' (1972). The movie depicts a process that is more barbaric than spiritual, leading many people to have a rather false view, and limited understanding of this most sacred of Lakota traditions. The similarity between the Sun Dance and a number of ceremonies from other cultures, such as fire walking, is that at a Sun Dance, the dancers dance for the people as a whole, for the health and well-being of the larger community.

The Sun Dance is a ceremony practised by several North

American Indian Nations, principally Plains Indians. Many of the ceremonies have local variations, but they share a number of common features, these include dancing, singing, drumming, and the experience of visions, fasting, and piercing. The Native American tribes who are known to have practised the Sun Dance are: The Arapaho, Arikara, Asbinboine, Cheyenne, Crow, Gros, Ventre, Hidutsa, Sioux, Plains Cree, Plains Ojibway, Sarasi, Omaha, Ponca, Ute, Shoshone, Kiowa, and Blackfoot tribes *(Walker, 1991)*.

Religious Ceremony

The Sun Dance was the most impressive, and important religious ceremony of the Plains Indians of 18th- and 19th-century North America, ordinarily held by the tribe once a year, usually at around the time of the Summer Solstice. During this period of time their buffalo hunting culture flourished, and the Sun Dance became the major annual communal religious ceremony. The dance was a celebration of the renewal of life, the spiritual rebirth of participants and their relatives. It was also a celebration of the regeneration of the living Earth (our Mother). The rituals involve personal sacrifice, and supplication to ensure harmony between all living beings, this continues in the modern day Sun Dances.

Thomas Mails (*1978*) writes, 'The Sun Dance includes every aspect of Sioux Religion, everything spiritual that they do on a year round basis is represented within the single ceremony.' (Sioux is a generic term used in the 19th and early 20th Century for the tribes that lived on the Plains of America. This has now been superseded by the traditional names of the tribes; however, it remains a generic term in many texts.)

The people who dance and those who attend to support the dancers believe that the sacred influences of the dance extend throughout the entire camp and last throughout the ceremony. They believe that awesome forces of good can be released in the

Sun Dance, which also means that its influence will expand and remain once the dance is over. All of this is in the minds of the traditional Plains peoples, and their increasing number of white Sun Dance supporters whenever a Sun Dance is held. I personally know several Sun Dancers, traditional Lakotas, Mexicans, and Whites who all hold this ceremony very dear and sacred. No one can attend a Sun Dance unless invited, and anyone who dances must prepare for a full year before they are allowed to dance. The Sun Dance is a profound celebration of thanksgiving, growth, prayer, and sacrifice. It is full of power, significance, and drama for the American Indians and all of mankind.

Michael Hull reports his own experience at his first Sun Dance (2000),

I sat in the rest arbor hoping to discover from somewhere enough strength to step back into the hocoka (the dance arena,) when the drum resumed its incessant pounding. My throat was parched. My skin was burned so badly it was blistered and starting to peel. My bare feet were cut, and bruised and bleeding.

I held in my hands two pins, two pieces of wood each about the size and shape of my little finger. One hour earlier, I was lying on a buffalo robe next to the sacred cottonwood tree that defined the middle of the arbor. I was biting down hard on a bundle of sage because Leonard Crow Dog had just cut holes in the flesh of my breast and stuck skewers through the holes. I tried to avoid wincing when I was led from the buffalo robe to a spot about eighty feet from the tree.

A 1/8th inch diameter sisal rope was tied to the top of the tree, and the other end was attached to a harness, which in turn was tied to my pins. I tried to pray while three thousand Lakota people watched me pull against the harness until my skin ripped as the skewers pulled through my flesh, while I was led back to the tree, and while the skin flaps were cut from my chest, wrapped in red fabric, and tied to the tree in an offering to the Great Spirit.

This very vivid account is reflected in the statements of other Sun Dancers that I know and have met. Another friend, James Dumshill tells me that he enters an ASC, assisted by the lack of food and water. He tells me that he focuses on praying for the people and for healing of the planet, becoming unaware of time and his surroundings for large amounts of time.

A good example of the healing that takes place at a Sun Dance was reported by Michael Hull (2000) at the first Sun Dance he led in Texas in 1998. A man called Rick attended; he had a little movement in his legs, and had been confined to a wheel chair for a year due to a degenerative condition in his back. Naturally, his legs had atrophied. On the third day of the dance, Rick was assisted out to the tree where he lay on the ground, as that was all he could do, and he prayed. A little later, he got up and walked rather haltingly out of the arbour. He gradually became able to walk a little better, until at the end of the day it was hard to imagine he had spent a year in a wheel chair.

Lakota Tradition

The Lakota name for the Sun Dance ceremony *is wiwanyag wacipi,* which means, 'They dance gazing at the sun.' The convocation is often brutal as participants dance barefoot for four days without any sustenance in the form of food and water. All the time they gaze at the sun and blow a whistle made from the ulna bone of the golden eagle. The ceremony is said to be a re-enactment of the White Buffalo Calf story (*Merrifield, 2006*).

Back in 1881, the United States government representatives on the reservations misinterpreted the Sun Dance, and caused the ceremony to be outlawed. It is now evident, however, that dances still continued out of the way of prying eyes until 1936, when the old laws were repealed. However, even after 1936, piercing continued to be prohibited. In his research, Thomas

Mails (1978) asked Frank Fools Crow about whether the piercing was ever fully terminated. He was told that at Pine Ridge the dances were held every year in one of two ways: as semipublic Sun Dances, without piercing, quietly done, with no fanfare, and with the occasional knowledge of agency officials, without any interference from them; or the secret Sun Dances with piercing, performed back in the hills.

The Sun Dance ceremony is performed in a large circle called either the Mystery Hoop or Circle. In the centre of this circle is a cottonwood tree that has been selected, and cut especially for the ceremony. This tree is often referred to as the Lodge Pole, Sacred Tree, or sometimes the Sun Pole. To the west of the tree is an altar, which comprises of a pipe rack and buffalo skull. Offerings are presented to the skull; the Cheyenne people stuff the eye and nose sockets with grass, representing bountiful vegetation for the buffalo, which in turn meant healthy buffalo for the people. In more recent times, the grass represented bringing the buffalo back to life, as the grass gave the animal life. The traditional Dakota believe that the bones of buffalo they have killed will rise again with new flesh. The soul was seen to reside in the bones of people and animals, and a skeleton is the equivalent of re-entering the womb of primordial life, a mystical rebirth.

Flags or stones are placed in the cardinal directions, east, west, north, and south, they also represent the limits of the circle. The spectators and supporters have the benefit of an arbour, which provides them with a sheltered area around the circumference of the circle. The entrance to the circle is through the east.

The sweat lodge ceremony is also an important part of the overall Sun Dance ceremony, and hence, one or more sweat lodges are created for each dance. These enable the participants to be purified before, and during the ceremony. Near the sweat lodge is a tipi where ceremonial items are kept, and where the participants dress.

Conducting the Sun Dance

In order to conduct a Sun Dance a number of people take on key roles. The person conducting the dance is sometimes called the Intercessor. This person acts as a channel through which communication with the Creator is possible. The Intercessor is always a holy or medicine man who is supported by other holy and medicine men. A medicine man is someone who practises healing. If he is both a priest and a medicine man, then he is known as a holy man. Consequently, the holy men are spiritual counsellors as well as healers. The holy man runs the entire ceremony, and instructs the participants in building the ceremonial tipi. He also provides direction to others, who gather the items required for the ceremony. Men known for their eminence in their community are selected to look for a cottonwood tree with a fork in the top. This is used for the first and centre pole of the lodge, otherwise known as the Sacred Tree, or Lodge.

The eldest woman of the camp usually leads a group of young women in ceremonial dress to the tree to remove its branches. The next morning, the moment the sun is seen over the eastern horizon, armed warriors charge the Lodge pole. They attack the tree in effort to symbolically kill it with gunshots and arrows. Once it is 'dead', it is cut down and taken to where the Sun Dance Lodge pole/Sacred Tree will be erected. Before raising the pole, a fresh buffalo head with a broad centre strip from the back of the hide and tail is fastened with strong throngs to the top crotch of the pole. Then, a special sacred bundle is placed on the fork. The Lakota people use a bundle containing brush, buffalo hide, long straws containing tobacco, and other ritual offerings. The pole is then raised, and set firmly in the ground, with the buffalo head facing toward the setting sun. This tree now symbolizes the centre of the world, connecting the heavens to the earth.

Each Sun Dance has a lead dancer who knows how to lead the dance ceremony. He is also responsible for building the ceremonial Lodge/Sacred Tree. The fork of the lodge represents the eagle's nest. The eagle plays a significant part in the Sun Dance, for it is one of the Plains Indians' most sacred animals. The eagle flies high, and is seen to be the creature that is closest to the Sun. Therefore; it is the link between man and spirit, the messenger that delivers prayers to the Creator (Wakan-Tanka).

In addition to being a messenger, the eagle also represents many human traits. The eagle is seen as courageous, swift, and strong. He has great foresight and knows everything. 'In an eagle there is all the wisdom of the world' (*Walker, 1991*). During the Sun Dance the eagle is the facilitator of communication between man and spirit, and works through the Intercessor. There are often other animal totems used throughout the ceremony. For instance, the Crow may be accompanied by a dancing eagle in his visions, with the eagle instructing him about the medicine acquired through the vision. During the Sun Dance a medicine man may use his eagle feather for healing, first touching the feather to the Lodge Pole, then to the patient, transferring the healing energy from the pole to the ill person.

It is the buffalo, however, that makes up the main theme of the Sun Dance. In various stories it was the buffalo that began the ritual. The Shoshone believe that the buffalo taught someone the proper way to carry out the dance, and the benefits of doing the dance. Buffalo songs, dances, and feasts commonly accompany the Sun Dance. The symbolic influence of the buffalo in the Sun Dance shows how important the animal was to the Plains Indians. It was the buffalo that symbolized life, for it was the buffalo that gave them their quality of life; food, clothing, shelters, and most of their utensils. These peoples' lives were intertwined with the buffalo's, and this important relationship was praised and blessed by the Sun Dance.

The buffalo has been incorporated in many ways in the Sun Dance. The Cheyenne hold a principle that all essential sacred items in the Sun Dance are related to the buffalo. The Lakota would sometimes place a dried buffalo penis against the Lodge Pole to give virility to the dancers. This reinforces the symbolic meaning of the ceremony as a celebration of the generative power of the sun.

The Dance Leader is always the first in line whenever the dancers assemble. At the end of each round, some of the dancers will present their pipes to the supporters in a sacred manner. The pipe is offered three times and refused. It is then accepted on the fourth occasion.

Traditionally, woman do not pierce, however, as more and more people have begun to Sun Dance some Dance Leaders do allow women to both dance and pierce. In all Sun Dances, women usually play an important role in the sweat lodges associated with the ceremony, often attending to the fire pit and providing the rocks and water needed for purification during the purification rituals.

Those who make vows to participate in the dance are known as pledgers. People pledge to dance for a certain number of years, usually four or multiples of four years, and consider their work incomplete until they have participated and sacrificed for the pledged number of years. In the Lakota tradition, participants are not referred to as Sun Dancers until they have completed their fourth year (*Hull, 2000*). They are then referred to as a completed dancer. The completed dancer can dance for additional years. Just as a four-year dancer has danced in each of the four directions (east, south, west and north); some people choose a full cycle of four years in each direction, a total of sixteen years.

Sometimes people participate in the Sun Dance as part of a Spirit Keeping ritual. This is a very old custom where the soul of a deceased person is 'kept' for up to a year before it is released at a Sun Dance ceremony, and allowed to make a full transition. Throughout the dance, singers and drummers lend their support to the dancers.

Piercing

The ritual piercing is conducted by the Dance Leader. He uses an awl, or a knife to penetrate the flesh of the chest, and creates two holes through which he places a stick or eagle claw. The eagle claw is then tied to a rope, the other end of which is attached to the Sacred Tree. The pledger then dances, and pulls back on the rope, often for many hours until the stick or claw finally breaks free as described by Michael Hull above. Prayers and songs are sung throughout this painful process to celebrate the bravery of those being pierced and expressing thanks for their sacrifice.

Sometimes a pledger will be pierced on their back, and one or two buffalo skulls attached to the piercings, which he then drags around the Mystery Circle until they break through the skin, releasing the skulls. This is considered a very great sacrifice, and only experienced pledgers will undertake such a task. Flesh offerings are also made; these are small bits of skin around a quarter of an inch square. These are cut from various parts of the body, usually the arms as sacrificial offerings of thanks to the Creator. Traditionally, women would participate in this part of the ceremony.

Duration

The Sun Dances last from four to eight days, the ceremony starts at sunset of the last day of preparation, and ends at sunset of the final day. It demonstrates continuity between life and death, regeneration. It shows that there is no true end to life, but a cycle of symbolic and true deaths and rebirths. The Sun Dancers believe that all of nature is interconnected, and dependent on one another, which symbolizes the fact that all living creatures are of equal importance in the cycles of life.

The number four is the prime sacred number for the Lakota, so a Sun Dance lasts four days, or two-times four days. Their belief system is that the Creator, or Great Spirit, (Wakan Tanka) created everything in fours, the four cardinal directions, four divisions of time, four parts in plants, and four periods in a human's life. Therefore, mankind can achieve harmony and completeness by arranging all of his ceremonies and activities in terms of this sacred number.

The Sun Dance also symbolizes a resolution with the conflict between being a people that views the buffalo as wise and powerful, even closer to the creator than humans, and having to kill and eat them to survive. Making the buffalo sacred, symbolically giving new life to it, and treating it with respect and reverence brings about a form of reconciliation. Without the buffalo, there would be death, and the Plains Indians saw that the buffalo not only provided them with physical well-being, but kept their souls alive too.

They also believed that buffaloes gave themselves readily for food. Therefore, as an act of reciprocity and gratitude, the natural course is to offer a part of themselves in return. Hence, the sacrifice of the dancers through fasting, thirst, and self-inflicted pain reflects the desire to return something of themselves to nature.

Piercing has also come to symbolize rebirth, it represents symbolic death, and resurrection. The Sun Dancer is therefore reborn, mentally and spiritually as well as physically, along with the renewal of the buffalo and the entire universe.

After the dancers all tear free, or after the end of the ceremony, the Sun Dance ends. The dancers are laid down on beds of sage to continue fasting and to share their visions with the holy man. These visions may hold new songs, new dance steps or even prophecies of the future. Whatever the outcome, the overall feeling for everyone present is of renewal and balance, the relationships between people and nature are once again reaffirmed.

Trance Dancing

Imagine darkness so intense and so complete covering you like a velvet blanket. A blackness that cuts you off from the everyday world, forcing you to draw deep into yourself, a blackness that makes you see with your heart instead of your eyes. You can't see, but your eyes seem open. You are isolated, but you know you are united with all living things. And out of darkness comes the roaring of the drums, the sound of the prayers. And among these sounds your ears catch the voices of the spirits, ghostlike, whispering to you from unseen lips. You feel the wings of birds brushing your face; feel the light touch of a feather on your skin. And always you hear the throbbing drums filling the empty space inside yourself, making you forget things that clutter your mind, making your body sway to their rhythm. Robbie Robertson (*Music for Native Americans,* 2004)

Any work on healing through ASC would not be complete without a brief discussion about trance dancing. It is often described as entering into our body – mind consciousness. My research led me to discover that since the beginning of recorded history dance has been used for the purpose of worshiping and healing. As with many indigenous practices this was, and continues to be, an expression of our connection to nature and an expression of God. The duplication or mimicking of nature through dance – sound and movement – was man's first and highest way of connecting with spirit (*Bougignion, 1973*) and was the origin of dance.

Trance dancing in its various forms is found in many cultures across the globe. Each continent has its own unique form of trance dancing based on the elements of nature, and various animals known to the local people. The purpose of these dances is to enter into the consciousness of, or become the spirit of the sun, the moon, and the various indigenous plants and animals. According to Wilbert Alix (2006), 'By dancing within the seclusion of darkness we discover parallel realities where solutions to seemingly unsolvable problems are possible.' In this way dance is seen as a doorway to the soul or 'spirit within', enabling the dancers to dance themselves into a state of trance (ASC) which enables them to connect to the healing powers of spirit. It is from these roots that trance dance has its origins.

Essentially, trance dancing is a unique blend of healing sounds, dynamic percussive rhythms, breathing processes, and the use of some form of a blindfold, which together create an ASC to promote emotional well-being, mental clarity, physical stamina, and for some, a spiritual awakening. I vividly remember visiting some friends one day, and playing a trance dance CD. The next day their young son said, 'Can you play that music again, the one that makes you dance?' He was expressing that which as adults we often fail to recognize, that music has a deep impact on our consciousness. The effect of the rhythmic beat of trance-dance music is quite profound. It is as if we allow ourselves to follow the music, it feels like it connects us to a part of ourselves that is very deep and very primal. As my friend's son implied, the music literally dances us.

Trance dancing is used to guide the participants on an inner journey, beyond the limitations of our usual perceptions into an ASC, out of our usual perceptions of time and space. It has been a part of shamanic and eastern dance cultures for millennia. Today, trance dance has become an increasingly popular way for people to enter an ASC for healing and transformation. Current teachers incorporate a number of modern day techniques such as using a bandana to cover our eyes. This assists in cutting out many of the major distractions of the brain, our outer vision by covering our eyes, and stimulates our inner vision, which enables us to have access to answers at a much deeper level of our existence.

According to Wilbert Alix (2006), the primary focus of trance dance is healing, and our relationship with spirit/God. Dancing in the seclusion of darkness enables us to enter an ASC, and to see new ways to overcome problems or resolve health issues. It is as if through trance dance we disappear, becoming more like spirit, and we hence dissociate from our problems, allowing us to release them completely. This enables us to develop a new sense of self, and to connect with the Universal Order.

The rhythm of the drum – know in many indigenous cultures as the heartbeat of mother earth – guides the dancers into a deep place of healing. By so doing, we are inviting spirit to dance through us, and to come to a place of peace with our true nature, experiencing the world through a lens of ecstasy.

Trance dance is used as a process of healing by the Whirling Dervishes of Turkey, the West African and Afro Brazilian cultures of the Candomble and Umbanda, as well as the Gnawa Moroccan tradition. The effect of these dances increases brain wave activity, heightens awareness, and moves the dancers, and musicians, into an ASC where healing and transformation can take place.

Essentially, through the dance, we communicate with our higher self and can bring about healing.

Chapter VI

In conclusion

My purpose in undertaking this research was to demonstrate the similarities of trance based healing found in many indigenous and modern peoples around the world. The exploration has been as fascinating as the processes have been diverse. However, one thing has become very apparent; no matter where I have been, or what literature I have read, there is one common theme. Someone, either the patient, and, or the healer, needs to go into an altered state of consciousness (trance) in order for a healing to occur. This altered state can be either a more 'up time' state such as in trance dancing or fire walking, or a 'down time' state, such as in hypnosis. Either way, normal every day consciousness needs to be changed in order for a healing to occur.

The journey I have undertaken has been fascinating and illuminating. I have travelled to various parts of the world where indigenous cultures maintain their close link with nature and continue their ancient traditions. I have also explored much of the scientific literature that is available and trained in various types of healing. I have discovered much, and yet I know there is far more to discover and understand than can be achieved in one lifetime.

I started this journey as a sceptic; however, as I started to explore, albeit tentatively, alternative ways of healing and the challenging of my model of the world, I began to see the seemingly infinite possibilities of healing methods around the globe. My own experiences with hypnosis, past life regression, Reiki, fire walking, plant medicine and so on, along with the reading and other research I have conducted, has led me to understand how far removed we are in the western world from that which is our natural heritage.

A lot of what I have discovered could be deemed to be subjective as there is little, if any, empirical or other scientific data to support these discoveries. However, I live in hope that over time new technologies will enable the accurate measurement of the phenomena described in this book, and indeed this is beginning in small and yet significant areas as scientists begin to push the boundaries of our perceived reality. The experiences I have had, and those I have shared with others have been very real to those of us who have participated, and they have opened me to a new way of being in the world.

One of the biggest problems facing the western world today is our frenetic way of life. We have forgotten that our purpose for being here is about being a human 'being', not a human 'doing'. And yet, the pace of life and drive for increasing material wealth has caused us to lose sight of our connection to nature and to others. This has caused me to bring into question what all of the consumer driven materialism means in a bigger context.

When I was a child I had a dream that I would train to be a doctor, and 'go out to America and help the Indian people'. I had a great sense of injustice and wanted to right some of the wrongs in the only way I knew how. Little did I know at the time, that as an adult, I would be turning to the indigenous ways to find solutions to some of the health problems of our modern world.

I have discovered, that the indigenous cultures in which I have worked and studied, have no incidences of mental illness, asthma, high blood pressure, cancers etc. So why would this be the case? It would be easy to fall into the romantic trap that some people create about indigenous cultures, thinking that we have to fully embrace their way of life if we are to 'save the world'. Of course we don't, and it would currently be almost impossible. However, the one thing they have that we certainly don't, is a sense of balance and working in harmony with each other and the world.

The !Kung (*Katz, 1984*), of the Kalahari are a good example of this. They have a system of bringing all types of imbalances back into equilibrium. All food is shared through a system based on fairness, the hunter keeping the prime parts and then distributing the remainder between their extended family, who in turn share with their family. This approach across all manner of daily activities, results in any disputes being resolved before they blow up. In this way, the people maintain a sense of equilibrium and balance. I have found variations of this system between all the indigenous cultures I have worked with. The other common theme has been in the various healing ceremonies.

In many of the cultures described in this book, healing ceremonies are created for the healing of the people as a whole. There may be one or two specific people who have asked to be healed; however, the ceremony is for the benefit of all. It may be through dance, plant medicine or some other means of entering into an altered state, but the purpose remains the same, it is for a healing, and for the greater good of the community.

Set out below are some of the questions I have asked myself as I have unravelled the complexities of healing through ASCs, along with my discoveries.

Question: How does healing occur?

I have cited many examples in the body of this book about different methods of healing; Hypnosis; Past Life Regression, Time Transformation Techniques and Shamanism; Shamanic Journeying, Shapeshifting; the Path of Pollen, Plant Medicine, Huna, Fire Walking, Sun Dancing and Trance Dancing. The first three, grouped under hypnosis, could arguably be seen as more modern ways of using ASC for healing, and those grouped under shamanism, the more ancient ways of healing. Yet all of these methods have a common thread; all require the healer or the patient (sometimes both) to go into an ASC for the healing and transformation to occur. This reminds me of the NLP (Neuro Linguistic Programming) adage that states that we cannot solve a problem with the same thinking that created the problem. Therefore, if applying this to dis-ease we cannot heal at the same level of consciousness at which we created the dis-ease.

Discovery 1: We cannot heal at the same level of consciousness as the level at which we create the dis-ease.

Question.2. What is the significance of the healer or the 'patient' going into an ASC?

My quest has led me to experience healings where the therapist or shaman guides a person, enabling him or her to go into a trance state for the healing to occur (hypnosis, PLR, TLT, fire walking), or, alternatively, whether the shaman/therapist goes into an ASC to facilitate the healing (soul retrieval and some plant medicine), or whether both shaman and patient go into an ASC (San Pedro, ayahuasca).

During my investigations, I have experienced and observed healings that occur either when the patient is guided into an ASC, or when the shaman goes into an ASC. I have also experienced healings when both myself, and the shaman have gone into trance (San Pedro and ayahuasca). In all of this, it appears that the single important factor is the intention; to heal. The difference between who goes into trance, and how this is achieved, is entirely subjective and largely irrelevant. Each method is a variation on a theme, and the theme is to enable a healing to occur.

I also know from personal experience with clients, that in order for me to work effectively as a hypnotherapist, I must also enter a different state of consciousness. My ASC may not be as deep as my client's, but I am definitely in an ASC rather than my usual up time awake state when I am doing this work.

Discovery 2: In order for healing to occur, it is irrelevant whether the patient or the therapist/ shaman goes into an ASC.

The importance is the intention to heal. The methods are merely ways of achieving the healing.

Question: Is it important whether the ASC is an 'up time' or a 'down time' state?

I have participated in, and led healing ceremonies in an 'up time' state such as fire walking and trance dancing, and have researched further into these. I have also conducted research into fire dancing.

In pursuit of a greater understanding, I have experienced the rise in energy as people go into heightened states of consciousness, and the massive energetic release that can occur on such occasions. It seems that as the energy rises, it gets to a point where the person knows at some level that they are ready to release the dis-ease, and so are ready to walk or dance on the fire. Once they arrive at the far end of the fire there is usually a sense of elation, along with a tremendous palpable release of energy. This sense of elation can last for some time, and then there is a desire to sleep. It is as if the body needs rest to realign itself fully.

I have worked with many people guiding them into 'down time' state in hypnosis, including past life regression and Time Line Therapy ™, and some shamanic journeying. I have also undertaken self-hypnosis and journeying, and have been guided by others. There are clearly different levels of down time states as discussed in the chapter on hypnosis. However, at each of these levels, I perceive a shift into a different level of consciousness and an allowing, which enables the healing to occur.

During an up time healing process, there is a sense of the energy building up to a crescendo to be released, whereas in a down time healing process, there is usually a relaxing sensation, thereby allowing a different type of release. Both processes work. These can be drawn as an energy continuum, where our normal state of consciousness is in the middle and we can move in either direction (which ever is our preference) to enable healing to occur.

Discovery 3: Healing occurs in both up time and down time states of consciousness.

The important point is that the state of consciousness is different from our normal waking state.

Question: Does the 'patient' need to be physically present?

For a number of healing processes it is important for the patient to be physically present. For example, in hypnosis, past life regression, Time Line Therapy, and soul retrieval, it is important for the patient to be present. This is because the patient plays an active role in these healing processes. In pure hypnosis as well as in PLR and TLT, the therapist guides the patient enabling them to go into the altered state in order to heal. In soul retrieval, the patient lays next to the shaman while he or she journeys to retrieve the soul part. The shaman can then breathe the retrieved 'part' into the patient. (This process is to my mind a shamanic variation of the NLP process of Parts Integration.) For these processes to work it is important for the patient to be present.

However, for a number of other healing processes it is not important for the patient to be present. I have cited examples in the main body of this book, such as, when the Maestro, Juan Navarro, worked with the teacher plant, San Pedro, to heal my husband several thousand miles away. I, along with many others have also undertaken distant healing processes with Reiki and prayer, with excellent results. In these cases the recipient does not need to know that others are working on their behalf.

One of my own clients has been suffering from a very rampant form of cancer. During our first session together he told me that he had first gone into remission about a month before we met. He is an eminent leader in the field of mental health, and had been surprised when he discovered that unbeknown to him, a group of people he didn't know very well had been meeting together to pray for him. The time they started to pray for him and the beginning of his remission coincided. He said that he had been so amazed that he had thought it may be worth trying some other therapies, and hence he made his way to my door.

The question all of this raises for me is: Is it a state of our current conditioning that we therapists feel the need for the patient to be present?

Discovery 4: The patient need not be present for healing to occur.

Question: Does a person need to actively participate in the process for healing to occur?

As discussed above, there are numerous anecdotes and personal stories that demonstrate the plausibility of people being prayed for and then a healing occurring. However, there are also examples of people being present and not participating in healing ceremonies who report being healed. An example of this is in fire walking ceremonies where people either choose not to walk, or are physically incapable of walking, yet they report 'spontaneous' healings.

One example is a lady, Anne, who came on one of my first fire walking programmes. She had very severe arthritis and told me that she would not be walking. I explained to her that this was ok and that she could still participate by being a part of the ceremony, helping to hold the energy so that others could walk safely. When we went out to the fire to begin the walk, she walked out with the group very slowly and tentatively due to the pain in her hips. We had a wonderful walk and everyone was elated as we walked back into the house for a light supper. I walked in behind everyone, and to my delight I saw Anne, walking along with the others with a huge grin on her face. The next morning she was exuberant as she told the group about her 'miraculous' healing despite not walking the fire. To my knowledge she remains pain free today, some six years on.

There are other examples of this discussed in the main body of the book where people have been healed simply by being present at a fire walk, or fire dance. It appears that the collective energy of the group and their intentions for healing is sufficient to enable other people present to heal.

Discovery 5: Being present at a healing ceremony is often enough for a healing to occur.

Question: What is the similarity or not, between hypnosis and other forms of healing through ASCs?

It is possible to measure the different levels of brain wave activity when people go into an ASC. However, there is a distinct lack of validated scientific evidence about the actual process of healing, the 'how'.

The similarities between hypnosis and these other types of healing is, that in all of these, one, or both, the healer and the patient must enter an altered state for the healing to occur. The second is the possibility of prestige suggestibility. In the western world when we are ill, it is the doctor we consult who is deemed to be in a position of prestige suggestibility or an authority figure. In my view, the same could be said for a shaman or healer in the indigenous cultures with which I have worked. He or she is in a position of 'power' or knowledge and hence their suggestions are likely to be accepted without question. The third similarity is that once a patient consults with a known hypnotherapist, shaman or therapist, there is usually an implicit assumption that they will receive some form of treatment, and hence a perceived assumption that in most cases they are willing to heal and go more easily into an ASC.

Discovery: The overt similarities between hypnotic type

therapies and shamanic type therapies are: an altered state of consciousness, prestige suggestibility and an implied willingness to heal.

Question: What has been my most important learning?

I have discovered something that had eluded me for some time. I can finally say that I understand the concept that time and space are irrelevant; they are merely constructs that help our conscious minds make sense of this reality we have created. This became so obvious to me when I was in Iquitos in the spring of 2008.

I had accepted the concept that time and space were constructs of our rational minds, but I had never had a deep knowing that this was true until the moment I spoke with my husband after my San Pedro experience with Juan Navarro. The fact that Juan knew nothing about me, and yet picked up the information about Robert who was several thousand miles away, was to my western mind, quite amazing. But what was even more amazing was the fact that the change in Robert was profound, immediate and enduring. I knew then without a doubt, that time and space are irrelevant in the true meaning of life.

Discovery 7: Time and space are mental constructs to help our conscious minds make sense of the world.

I have experienced many incidents of healing both as a patient and a 'healer'. However, I have come to realize that whilst I would love to be able to produce validated evidence of these various healing methodologies, there is very little available. We do not have the technology yet to be able to demonstrate what happens during these healings, nor how these various healings occur.

It seems to me, that all we can do is gather more and more evidence of healings occurring and attempt to find the commonalities between them all. My hope is that if we continue to collect as much information as we can, we will one day have the instruments to measure the processes effectively. People in the western world predominately like to 'know' that this is the way to do something. Whereas, I have come to realize that there are many ways to climb the mountain, but at the end of the day the important thing is that we get there. It is actually irrelevant how we choose to get there.

A Final Word

In 2002, 82-year old Don Ramon came down from the Andes in Peru to my home in order to bring his methods of healing and knowledge to the western world. He came because he had been 'told' long ago that the day would come when the western world was ready to learn and to heal. The day came and he travelled thousands of miles to share this knowledge with those of us who are willing to learn. He came, not so we would completely abandon our ways of life, but to enable us to blend the best of the modern world with the best of the ancient.

Through the research I have done into altered states of consciousness and their role in healing, I am convinced that Don Ramon was right. We can blend the best of both worlds to create an approach to life and healing that allows us to use the spectrum of consciousness to raise our awareness and hence our ability to heal ourselves and the world around us.

References

Journal articles

Dorrance, David, MD. *Effects of peyote on human chromosomes.* Journal of the AMA 1975, vol 234, No.3 Oct.

Books

Achterberg, Jeanne, (1991) *Imagery in healing: Shamanism and modern medicine.* Shambala Publications Inc.

Andreas, Steve & Andreas, Connirae, (1988). *Change your mind and keep the change.* Real People Press.

Sun Bear, & Wabun, (1987). *The path of power.* Simon & Schuster Ltd.

Bentov, Itzhak, (1988). Stalking the wild pendulum: On the mechanics of consciousness. Inner Traditions Bear & Co.

Barber, J., (1996) Hypnosis and suggestion in the treatment of pain. Norton Professional Books

Bruce, Eve, (2002) *Shaman MD.* Destiny Books

Burkan, Tolly, (2004). Extreme spirituality: Radical approaches to awakening. Council Oak Books.

Buxton, Simon, (2004). The shamanic way of the bee: Ancient wisdom and healing practices of the bee masters. Destiny Books.

Cade, C. Maxwell & Coxhead, Nona, (1987). The awakened mind; Biofeedback and the development of higher states of awareness. Element Books Ltd.

Cannon, Alexander, (1954). The power within: The re-examination of certain psychological and philosophical concepts in the light of recent investigations and discoveries. Rider and Co.

Carrel, Alexis, (1961). *Man the unknown.* MacFadden Publications.

Carver, Jonathon, (1802). *Travels in North America.* Publisher unkown.

Coelho, Paulo (1999). The pilgrimage: A contemporary quest for ancient wisdom. Thorsons.

Crasilneck, Harold & Hall, James (1985) *Clinical hypnosis: Principles and applications.* Grune and Stratton

Crow Dog, Leonard & Erdoes, Richard, (1996). *Crow Dog: Four generations of Sioux medicine men.* Harper Collins, Australia.

Danforth, Loring M., (1989). Firewalking and religious healing: Anastenaria of Greece and the American firewalking movement. Princeton University Press.

Dobkin de Rios, Marlene, (1990). *Hallucinogens: Cross cultural perspectives.* Prism Unity.

Einstein, Albert, (1996). *Relativity: The special and general theory.* Crown Publications.

Eliade, Mircea, & Trask, Wilard, (1989). *Shamanism, Archaic techniques of ecstasy.* Arkana Books.

Elman, Dave (1964). *Hypnotherapy.* Westwood Publishing Co.

Evans, Schultes, Richard, (1972). Flesh of the Gods: An overview of hallucinogens in the western hemisphere. Arkana Books.

Evans, Schultes, Richard and Hoffman Albert, (1982). *Plants of the gods: Their sacred and hallucinogenic powers.* Inner Traditions Bear & Co.

Everett, Daniel, (2008). *Don't sleep, there are snakes.* Profile Books Ltd.

Freedom Long, Max, (1999). *What Jesus taught in secret.* De Vorss & Co.

Greenfield, Susan, (2002). *The private life of the brain.* Penguin.

Grob, Charles, (2003). *Hallucinogens: A reader.* Jeremy P. Tarcher.

Hall, L. Michael (1996). *Meta states: A domain of logical levels.* International Society of Neuro-semantics.

Hammerschlag, Carl, (1988). *The dancing healers.* Turtle Island Press.

Harner, Michael, (1973). *Hallucinogens and shamanism.* Oxford University Press Inc. U.S.

Harner, Michael, (1992). *The way of the Shaman.* Harper San

Francisco

Heaven, Ross & Charing, Howard G., (2006). *Plant medicine.* Destiny Books, U.S.

Hebb, Donald O, (2002). The organisation of behaviour: A neurophysiological theory. Lawrence Erlbaum Associates Inc.

Heyoka, Merrifield, (2006). *Eyes of Wisdom.* Beyond Worlds Publishing.

Hull, Michael, (2001). *Sun dancing: A spiritual journey on the red road.* Inner Traditions Bear & Co.

Inge Heinze, Ruth, (1984). Trance and healing in Southeast Asia today: Twenty-one case studies. Unknown Binding.

Ingerman, Sandra, (2006). Soul Retrieval: Mending the fragmented self. Harper One.

James, William, (2003). The will to believe and other essays in popular philosophy. Dover Publications Inc.

James, Tad & Woodsmall, Wyatt (1989). *Time line therapy and the basis of personality.* Meta Publications.

Johnson, Dorothy, (1974). *A man called Horse.* Ballantine Books.

Katz, Richard, (1984). Boiling energy: Community healing among the Kalahari Kung! Harvard University Press.

King, Serge Kahili. (1990). *The Urban Shaman.* Simon & Schuster.

Klein, Melanie & Mitchell, Juliet (1987). *The selected Melanie Klein.* The Free Press.

Kroger, William S., & Fezler, William D, (1978). *Clinical and experimental hypnosis: Imagery condictioning.* Lipincott, Williams and Wilkins

Lafferty, Lavedi, & Hollowell, Bud (1983). *Eternal dance: There is no life after death, there is no death.* Llewellyn Publications.

Lawlor, Robert, (1994). Voices of the first day: *Awakening the in aboriginal dreamtime.* Inner Tradition Bear & Co.

Lawrence, Allen & Lisa, (1994). Huna: Ancient miracle healing practices and the future of medicine. Login Publishers Consortium.

Le Cron, Lesley, (1964). *How to stop smoking through self hypnosis.* Wilshire Book Co.

Libet, Benjamin, (2004). Mind Time: The temporal factor in consciousness. Harvard University Press.

Lilly, John, (1985). The centre of the cyclone: Looking into inner space. Ronin Publishing

Mails, Thomas, E, (new edition 1998). *Sundancing at Rosebud and Pine Ridge.* Council Oak Books.

Matthews, John, (1991). *The Celtic Shaman: A practical guide.* Rider & Co

McKenna, Terence, (1999). Food of the Gods: A radical history of plants, drugs and human evolution. Rider & Co.

McKinney, Laurence O, (1994) *Neurotheology: Virtual religion in the 21st century.* American Institute for Mindfulness

Morgan, Dylan, (2003). *Hypnosis for beginners.* Cosmo Publications.

Mount, Guy, (1993). The peyote book: A study of native medicine. Peyote Press.

Narby, Jeremy, (1999). The cosmic serpent: DNA and the origins of knowledge. Phoenix.

Narby, Jeremy, (2006). *Intelligence in nature.* Jeremy P. Tarcher

New King James Version, (2007). *Holy Bible.* Nelson Bibles.

Neeley, Bill, (2007). The life and times of the last Comanche chief: Quanah Parker. Castle Books.

Newburg, Andrew, D'Aquili, Eugene D & Rause, Vince (2001). *Why God won't go away: Brain Science and the biology of belief.* Ballantine Books Inc.

Overdurf, John & Silverthorn, Julie (1994). *Training Trances: Multi-level communication in therapy and training.* Metamorphous Press, US. 3rd edition.

Overdurf, John & Silverthorn, Julie (1998). *Dreaming Realities.* Crown House Publishing.

Penfield, Wilder, (1978). Mystery of the Mind: A critical study of consciousness and the human brain. Princeton University

Press.

Perkins, John, (1994). The world is as you dream it: Shamanic teachings form the Amazon. Inner Traditions Bear & Co.

Perkins, John, (1997). Shapeshifting: Techniques for global and personal transformation. Inner Traditions Bear & Co.

Persinger, Michael (1987). *Neuropsychological bases of God beliefs.* Greenwood Press.

Pert, Candace, (1999). Molecules of emotion: Why you feel the way you feel. Pocket Books

Rhawn, Joseph ,(1992). The right brain and the unconscious: Discovering the stranger within. Perseus Books. U.S.

Schultes, Richard E., (1992). Plants of the Gods: Their sacred healing and hallucinogenic powers. Inner Traditions Bear and Co.

Simeona, Morrnah K, (1980) *Ho'opnonpono notes.* Huna Research Inc.

Steiger, Brad, (1982). *Kahuna magic.* Whitford Press, U.S.

Targ, Russell & Ketra Jane (1999). Miracles of Mind: Exploring nonlocal consciousness and spiritual healing. New World Library.

Tart, Charles, (2000). *States of consciousness.* Universe.com

Tomlinson, Andy, (2006). Healing the eternal soul: Insights into past life regression. O Books.

Van der Post, Laurens, (new edition 2002). *The lost world of the Kalahari.* Vintage Books.

Wagner McClain, Florence (1986). *A practical guide to past life regression.* Llewellyn Publications.

Walker, James & Demaillie, Raymond, (1991). *Lakota belief and ritual.* University of Nebraska Press.

Walkington, David L, (1960). *Economic Botany.* Malki Museum Press.

Weiss, Brian, (1994). *Many lives, many masters.* Piatkus Books

Weiss, Brian (2004). *Same soul, many bodies.* Piatkus Books

Wesselman, Hank (2011) *The Bowl of Light.* Sounds True

Wolberg, Lewis, (2007). Medical hypnosis V1. The principles of hypnotherapy. Kessinger Publishing.

Zemlicka, Shannon & Kudson, Shannon, (2004). *Quanah Parker*. Lerner Publications.

Internet

Cadigan, Ken, *Firewalking*. Retrieved from www.kencadigan. com 12th August 2008.

Dylan, Peggy (2002). *A brief history of fire walking*. Retrieved from www.sundoor.com on 11th July 2008.

Fehmi, Les. (2007) *The open focus brain: Harnessing the power of attention to heal mind and body*. Retrieved from www. openfocus.com 15th September 2008.

Freedom Long, Max, (1955). *Huna Bulletin: Growing into light*. Retrieved October 16th 2008.

Freedom Long, Max, (1961). *Letters on Huna, Mana #4*. Retrieved October 16th 2008.

Marsolek, Patrick, *How valuable are altered states of consciousness?* Retrieved from www.innerworkingresources.com October 21st 2008.

Meijan, Tim, (2006). *An interview with Wilbert Alix*. Retrieved from www.trancedance.com on 2nd October 2008.

Past life regression definition. Retrieved from www.wikipaedia. com 16th September 2008.

WHO (World Health Organisation), www.who.int. Retrieved statistics 8th Sept 2008.

BOOKS

O-BOOKS

SPIRITUALITY

O is a symbol of the world, of oneness and unity; this eye represents knowledge and insight. We publish titles on general spirituality and living a spiritual life. We aim to inform and help you on your own journey in this life.

If you have enjoyed this book, why not tell other readers by posting a review on your preferred book site? Recent bestsellers from O-Books are:

Heart of Tantric Sex
Diana Richardson
Revealing Eastern secrets of deep love and intimacy to Western couples.
Paperback: 978-1-90381-637-0 ebook: 978-1-84694-637-0

Crystal Prescriptions
The A-Z guide to over 1,200 symptoms and their healing crystals
Judy Hall
The first in the popular series of six books, this handy little guide is packed as tight as a pill-bottle with crystal remedies for ailments.
Paperback: 978-1-90504-740-6 ebook: 978-1-84694-629-5

Take Me To Truth
Undoing the Ego
Nouk Sanchez, Tomas Vieira
The best-selling step-by-step book on shedding the Ego, using the
teachings of *A Course In Miracles*.
Paperback: 978-1-84694-050-7 ebook: 978-1-84694-654-7

The 7 Myths about Love...Actually!
The journey from your HEAD to the HEART of your SOUL
Mike George
Smashes all the myths about LOVE.
Paperback: 978-1-84694-288-4 ebook: 978-1-84694-682-0

The Holy Spirit's Interpretation of the New Testament
A course in Understanding and Acceptance
Regina Dawn Akers
Following on from the strength of *A Course In Miracles*, NTI
teaches us how to experience the love and oneness of God.
Paperback: 978-1-84694-085-9 ebook: 978-1-78099-083-5

The Message of A Course In Miracles
A translation of the text in plain language
Elizabeth A. Cronkhite
A translation of *A Course in Miracles* into plain, everyday
language for anyone seeking inner peace. The companion
volume, *Practicing A Course In Miracles*, offers practical lessons
and mentoring.
Paperback: 978-1-84694-319-5 ebook: 978-1-84694-642-4

Thinker's Guide to God
Peter Vardy
An introduction to key issues in the philosophy of religion.
Paperback: 978-1-90381-622-6

Your Simple Path
Find happiness in every step
Ian Tucker
A guide to helping us reconnect with what is really important in
our lives.
Paperback: 978-1-78279-349-6 ebook: 978-1-78279-348-9

365 Days of Wisdom
Daily Messages To Inspire You Through The Year
Dadi Janki
Daily messages which cool the mind, warm the heart and guide
you along your journey.
Paperback: 978-1-84694-863-3 ebook: 978-1-84694-864-0

Body of Wisdom
Women's Spiritual Power and How it Serves
Hilary Hart
Bringing together the dreams and experiences of women across
the world with today's most visionary spiritual teachers.
Paperback: 978-1-78099-696-7 ebook: 978-1-78099-695-0

Dying to Be Free
From Enforced Secrecy to Near Death to True Transformation
Hannah Robinson
After an unexpected accident and near-death experience, Hannah
Robinson found herself radically transforming her life, while a
remarkable new insight altered her relationship with her father, a
practising Catholic priest.
Paperback: 978-1-78535-254-6 ebook: 978-1-78535-255-3

The Ecology of the Soul
A Manual of Peace, Power and Personal Growth for Real People
in the Real World
Aidan Walker
Balance your own inner Ecology of the Soul to regain your
natural state of peace, power and wellbeing.
Paperback: 978-1-78279-850-7 ebook: 978-1-78279-849-1

On the Other Side of Love
A Woman's Unconventional Journey Towards Wisdom
Muriel Maufroy
When life has lost all meaning, what do you do?
Paperback: 978-1-78535-281-2 ebook: 978-1-78535-282-9

Practicing A Course In Miracles
A Translation of the Workbook in Plain Language and With
Mentoring Notes
Elizabeth A. Cronkhite
The practical second and third volumes of The Plain-Language
A Course In Miracles.
Paperback: 978-1-84694-403-1 ebook: 978-1-78099-072-9

Readers of ebooks can buy or view any of these bestsellers by
clicking on the live link in the title. Most titles are published
in paperback and as an ebook. Paperbacks are available in
traditional bookshops. Both print and ebook formats are
available online.

Find more titles and sign up to our readers' newsletter at
http://www.johnhuntpublishing.com/mind-body-spirit

Follow us on Facebook at https://www.facebook.com/OBooks/
and Twitter at https://twitter.com/obooks